# NOBLE LETTERS

*to creative*

# NURSES

**COLOURING THE IMAGE OF THE NURSING PROFESSION**

## ISRAELMORE AYIVOR

# NOBLE LETTERS to CREATIVE NURSES

**Israelmore Ayivor**

**NOBLE LETTERS
TO CREATIVE NURSES**
Copyright © *2017* – Israelmore Ayivor.



Facebook: Israelmore Ayivor
Twitter: @IsraelmoreA
Instagram: @israelmore.ayivor

I write, I speak and I blog on personal development, self-discovery and I help young people to kick start to live their dreams. To book me for your conference or workshop as a resource person, contact me;

Email: israelmoreayivor@gmail.com
Phone: +233244920845 or +233209060903

# ACKNOWLEDGEMENT

God is good. Glory be unto His name for great things He has done. Greater things He will do. I am specially thankful to Him for His guidance over my life.

I am deeply grateful to my mother, Precious Nutornutsi who happened to be my first teacher and nurse. The greatest cares I have ever received came from her. I'm also grateful for the anonymous nurses who cared for me since I was a child. My mother's narrative about my childhood life informed me of a certain nurse who once cared for me when I was severely ill. She could not find my veins after many trials and had to resort to serious prayers for few minutes. Just after the prayer, the veins became visible and there she was, happy and grateful to God for saving a life. I may not know you, sister, but the care of God through you sustained me. May you and your generations be blessed!

To all tutors who trained me in the Nursing Training College; Sister Josephine Ansu-Gyeabour, Rev. Sister Constantia Atachie, Mr. Paul Worlasi Kokuma, Mr. Emmanuel Mawuena, Sister Bella Johnson, Sister Ernestina Noi, Sister Patience Senaya, Sister Epiphania Sepenu, Mr. Dordzi Wilson, Mr. Mawuli Tetegah, Mr. Samuel MacCarthy, Mr. Frank Agbo, Mr. Paul Attipoe, Sister Patience Doe, Sister Patience Dotsey, Sister Ruth Kumahor, and others. You have instilled into my colleagues and I deeper roots of knowledge and skills we can never pay you for. May you and your generations be rewarded.

I am highly indebted to the 2010/2011 team of SRC Executives of Ho NTC among who I served as a General Secretary. I shaped my skills in leadership and writing while I served among you. Todzoh Emmanuel, you have been one of the most effective and monumental SRC Presidents I know. I am proud of the unique Diploma Group 11 batch. Time spent with you guys was one of the most remarkable memories I shall always remember for the rest of my life.

To all my friends and mates at University of Health and Allied Sciences, and to my lecturers; Mr Agbezorli, Mr. George Bandji Tesilimi, Mr. Benjamin Amoako, Mrs. Belinda Adzimah-Yeboah, Madam Comfort Worna Lotse and others that I may not mention here. I trust your experiences and believe you are producing the nurses the nation and the world needs at large. Rev. Sister Constantia Atachie, I am excited to be your student once again. I specially acknowledgement you Professor Mwini-Nyaledzigbor Prudence Portia, professor extraordinaire and to Dr. Judith Anaman-Torgbor, my research supervisor.

Finally to the hardworking staff and former staff of Keta Municipal Hospital (KMH), I say Ayeekoo. I appreciate every single moment of working with you, learning much from you and sharing the little I know with you. May you keep doing the good work you have never been tired of doing. To the Nurse Managers I met since I started working at KMH; Sister Margaret Gbadrive, Sister Florence Akussah and currently, Sister Constance Korkpa and Sister Bridget Kusse. Our Doctors, Dr. Asare Bediako, Dr. Michael Nii Hammond, Dr. Ernest Boakye and others. Specially to Dr. Murtala Antaro, Mr. Sylvester Thompson, Edem Akakpo and Sromawuda Boni, I still remember how supportive you were during my first book launching ceremony.

A special acknowledgment to my big brother, friend and senior in the nursing profession, Mr Brempong Richard, the former President of Nurses Christian Fellowship (2009/2010) of Ho NTC and Mr. Isaac Dzubey. Your timely intervention saved me through the nursing training college at a very crucial time and I will remember this for the rest of my life.

Finally, to my biological siblings; Michael Akpenyo Ayivor, Hawa Melinawo Ayivor and others. I am grateful to have you around. I see hope building up as we grow as a family. The future is bright; God is making it brighter!

# DEDICATION

This book is dedicated to

*Nana Sarah Yeboah, the CEO and Founder of Sangy Nursing Services, Co—founder and Vice-President of The Sangy Foundation and Senior Staff Nurse at Ridge Hospital, Accra. You are a "nurse extraordinaire". Your contribution to the growth of Africa is outstanding. Keep it up dear. Do more for God, community, country and continent!*

*Mrs. Belinda Adzimah-Yeboah, a lecturer at University of Health and Allied Sciences. You have truly inspired to add a great volume of knowledge on legal matters pertaining to my profession. The knowledge I acquired, I promised to share and that has been the reason for chapter five of this book. God bless you.*

*Professor Prudence Portia Mwini-Nyaledzigbor, the Dean of School of Nursing & Midwifery, University of Health and Allied Sciences, Ho. Students' concerns are your heart beart. You are a down-to-earth leader.*

*The Federal SRC President of UHAS (2017-2018), Master Derrick Asare and his team of leaders.*

*All Executives of Ghana Nurses And Midwives Association (GRNMA) at National, Regional, District and Station levels. More grease to your elbows!*

# TABLE OF CONTENTS

# FOREWORD BY MR PAUL KOKUMA

Nurses are just like farmers. They work just like farmers do. The farmer wants to prevent pests from attacking his animals and crops; nurses want to prevent infections from worsening the health of their patients. While farmers add fertilizers to promote the yields of crops, nurses give medications to promote the health of patients. Farmers are at risks of many dangers while working hard to achieve their aims; nurses are not different; their risks are in multiples of what they already know.

It is a blessing to take care of a fellow man. It is a privilege to care for someone who can't be able to care for himself. Above all, it is good news to offer education to someone concerning a health condition; and education that will go a long way to prevent illness in the future.

An in-patient has the privilege of having a sky-wide access to the nurse 24 hours each day. It means, nurses are the closest health workers a patient can find. The closest person has the best information and skills and the best information and skills provide the best solution to problems be it actual or potential. In the book "House Rules", Jodi Picoult wrote, *"If you really want to get the answers to a question about court, you should spend more time buttering up the clerks than the judges. It's like nurses in the hospital tend to know more than the doctors most of the time"*. Yes! Everyone in the hospital team must know, but Nurses should know best. But is that the reality in our hospitals, clinics and health centres? I leave the reader to make his/her conclusions.

However, if you feel like the pale colour of the image of nursing needs recolouring, the paint is in your hands.

It is a great pleasure to have this book published by one of my students, Israelmore Ayivor who is passionate about sharing good information through publishing. This book, I believe caries the colours and brushes to paint good images about our noble profession, nursing. In other words, it has the eraser to clean the bad image already existing, obviously known to you. Most of the knowledge shared in the contents of this book, you're about to meet them for the first time in your life. However, some are things you already know during your school days, but perhaps because of the length of time, you have forgotten and need to be refreshed. The refresher is in these "Noble Letters" and you will love to refill your memory again and again.

The bundles of researches conducted to enrich the contents of this book make the book to standout not just for nursing, but for anyone in any field who wants to know some deeper things about what nurses do.

If we are talking about creating a better nursing reputation in Ghana, Africa and beyond, nursing students should be the main focus. I am excited about the chapter of this book that focuses on Nursing Students with the intention of inculcating in them the ability to maintain their humble, innocent, sober, calm, positive and undefiled attitudes even with the change in time. I recommend that every nursing student grabs a copy of this book read it, and take it as a guide to match his or her times during the training days.

Another unique thing about this book is the inspirational poems which have inspired me so much, touching on the work of the nurses; what they do and what they should do. The experiences shared here are real. The theories are helpful and worth reading again and again. This book again treats briefly legal concerns and put nurses on their toes to act right and professionally to avoid committing costly mistakes, thereby washing the reputation of nursing in muddy waters. It is my wish that all nurse managers advice their nurses to get their copies of this book to get informed and inspired. When a nurse grabs, reads and apply the knowledge compiled in this masterpiece, a big chunk of the anxiety of the nurse managers will be relieved since the book acts as an inspirer, informer, attitude shaper, intent amender and behaviour corrector.

**Mr. Paul Worlasi Kokuma**
**(Principal Heath Tutor, Ho Nurses Training College)**

# PRAISES FOR THE "NOBLE LETTERS"

"Noble letters", is a fantastic book. The contents are powerful. It is highly recommended for every nurse. It is a must read. Well done, Mr Ayivor." – **Naomi Arthur,** *Nursing Tutor, Nurses Training College, Ho.*

This is a remarkable book about the future of nursing and midwifery. "Noble Letters" is the first book that brings out the realities of nursing and midwifery practice. A must read. – **Paul Worlasi Kokuma**, *Principal Health Tutor, Ho Nursing Training College.*

This is a wonderful masterpiece, full of heart balms to nurses worldwide. After reading and contemplating on the words in this book, I am super inspired to give out my best for humanity no matter how unfavourable the conditions are. I say bravo to the writer for a beautiful job done. "Noble Letters" is a highly recommended book for nurses. – **Esther Adegah,** *University of Health and Allied Sciences, Ho.*

You have in your palm a handbook well prepared to motivate you even through your stress period and still achieve your nursing goals. It encourages the nurse to build motivation within him/herself for the sacrificial work. Every nurse must have a copy and read it once a while. – **Linda Kuffour,** *Keta Municipal Hospital.*

Books are written to inform, reform, inspire and to rebuke. Apostle Paul's letter to churches has contributed to building the body of Christ. I think this book carries enough "nursing epistles" to nurse the sick image of nursing and brighten the profession in the eyes of pessimists. I think the writer; Israelmore Ayivor did a fantastic job exposing facts to be our guide. – **Nash Abigail**, *Nurses and Midwifery Training School, Ashanti Mampong.*

There are so many books that can correct behaviour and inspire individuals to give out their best. "Noble Letters" is one of them. It is found on the concept of rebuilding the passion in the nurse to work hard and redeem the image of the profession. – **Josephine Bensah**, *Nursing and Midwifery Training College, Keta*

The orderly representation of the contents of this book is just wonderful. Each of the letters in this book will serve a purpose of transforming the mindset of the reader to ensure nursing has a clean image. – **Nancy Danso.** *– Narh Bitah Nurses Training School*

Nurses need to be reminded and encouraged to give out their bests. This is what "Noble Letters" is about. The image of nursing at large I hope will be cleansed when pieces of information shared here are put into practice by Nurses and Student Nurses. – **Mercy Senehia**, *Phronesis Health & Development.*

I know the image of Nursing is falling, especially in our diaspora. I have gathered a great load of information here, inspiring me not to forget that we hold in our own hands the tool to lift up the falling image. – **Obaa Rosemary**, *Manso Amenfi Health Centre.*

I have read so many books, but I see "Noble Letters" standing tall among them. This book speaks about real situations pertaining to the nursing profession, and inspires the reader (being a nurse or not) to understand what nurses go through day in, day out. This book is also functional when it comes to attitude building for nurses and I seriously recommend it for everyone especially nurses and student nurses. – **Adelaide Yeboah,** *Nursing and Midwifery Training College, Keta*

You have done a marvelous job, Mr. Ayivor. If no book at all, all nurses should read this book and I believe Nursing will regain its identity. It contains information to show nurses right directions. Thank you very much. – **Asirifi Isaac Gunu,** *University of Health and Allied Sciences, Ho.*

The book "Noble Letters" is very interesting. It advices Student Nurses not to allow experience and time to change their characters. I recommend it as a must read for every nurse irrespective of their ranks or levels of education. – **Bridget Ama Serwaa Ganah**, *Integrated College of Allied Health and Nursing, Obuasi.*

"Noble Letters" by the motivational guru, Israelmore Ayivor has motivated me to maintain and improve my character irrespective of my experiences. Together, I believe when the information shared here are put into use, Nursing as a profession will earn a great reputation than ever before. – **Mirinda Kudzu Lumorsi**, *Nursing Training College, Techima-Krobo*

Israelmore Ayivor's 25 books are just fantastic. "Noble Letters" is another mind blowing collection of knowledge shared to ensure that the nurse takes caution and work hard to redeem the image of her (his) profession. **– Rebecca Adwoa Mensah**, *Nursing Training College, Ho.*

This is an impressive book, specially written to correct wrong behaviours and also inspire nurses to love their profession. Having gone through, I enjoyed the diction and I recommend it for all nurses and student nurses. **– Ruby Narh Padiki**, *Nursing and Midwifery Training College, Keta*

Having gone through the book "Noble Letters", I learnt that nurses should be inspired by the work they do, but not by the "thank you" from patients and their relatives. This will help balance their emotions towards work. **– Georgina Agonyo,** *Nursing Training Collage, Pantang*

I learnt so many things in this book, but the most significant that I will keep in my heart is "Caring is the heart of Nursing". I promise to be part of the change that the letters in this book advocates. **– Cantil Jennifer,** *Nyaniba Health College, Tema.*

Reading this book has offered me another chance to update myself concerning the ethical issues relating to my work as a nurse. I have also acquired much information to inspire myself and continue contributing my quota to improving the image of nursing. **– Martha Akuffo,** *Keta Municipal Hospital*

Israelmore, God bless you for this wonderful letters. They are like the Epistles of Apostle Paul to the nations to help correct their behaviours. The name of our profession will shine when we lift our hands to pick up the right attitude and build worthy relationships during the course of our work. – **Richard Attitsogbui,** *Nursing and Midwifery Training College, Keta*

Nursing is an art and a nurse must be creative in order to ensure her nursing goals are achieved. The book "Noble Letters" is a great contribution towards inspiration and creativity in the nursing profession. I call on Practicing and Student Nurses to use the information provided here to raise the standard of the noble profession**. – Jennifer Adikah,** *Midwifery Training School, Hohoe.*

It is so pathetic that the noble tag on our profession (nursing) has been scraped off for many reasons. However, there is a chance and there is also more hope for illumination which "Noble Letters" has given birth to. This book is here for massive transformation. I salute you, Mr Ayivor**. – Esther Adzato,** *Nursing Training Collage, Ho.*

Going through the pages of this book alone made me to "rethink" about my career. It is amazing and I felt fulfilled having carried many cautions here. I encourage my dear colleague nurses to read this noble letter. It will make you see Nursing the way you have not seen it before. – **Nice Kludzi,** *Nursing and Midwifery Training College, Keta.*

I see this book as a source of very useful information that can transform the attitude of nurses and midwives by reminding them of the roles they have been trained to play. I believe it was truly written to correct specific things and thereby make nursing an attractive profession as it used to be. I recommend it for all nurses and midwives practicing and schooling. – **Gladys Hunkpor,** *Pentecost University College.*

I think "Noble Letters" has come at the right time at the right time, especially when the public constantly complains of poor nursing services rendered by some nurses. It contains series of reminders to put nurses on their toes to redeem the falling image of the profession whose integrity we have vowed to uplift. – **Catherine Ahiagbe,** *Nursing and Midwifery Training College, Keta.*

There is so much knowledge this book carries. It is a must read for nurses. From this book, I learnt a lot to guide my school life now and career life later on. It reminds me of things I already know and informs me on things I am yet to know about nursing. – **Elta Gbedzo,** *Nursing and Midwifery Training College, Kumasi.*

This book is very educative, motivational and contains what the nurse and the nursing student needs to give out his/her best. I am convinced it was carefully written to give a reminder to all personnel in the nursing profession. – **Fortune Ahiale,** *Nursing and Midwifery Training College, Lawra.*

I just love the words of caution in this masterpiece. I hope many books like type will soon get published to help inform and re-inform nurses to give out their bests while they practice. – **Justine Ahedor,** *Nursing and Midwifery Training College, Kete-Krachi*

Israelmore has compiled a fantastic book for nurses. But I think, this book is not only good for nurses. Portions of this book are relevant to all health workers. With the contents found here, I know this book will not leave the reader the same. There will be definitely a change in attitude positively in anyone who is determined to start, continue and finished reading this book. – **Victoria Agbezuke,** *College of Health, Kintampo.*

I read this book during my first week as a midwifery student while orientation was on-going for us. This book offered me the opportunity to prepare my mind ready for my first midwifery class. I believe it is a great informer compiled by my brother who never likes to hide good information from people who need it. – **Hawa Melinawo Ayivor,** *Nursing and Midwifery Training College, Keta.*

This book contains great pieces of helpful information put together through constructive researches and rich experiences of a great writer and an experienced nurse. It throws a deeper light on the art of caring by the nurse and how the nurse on the job can manage tendencies of frustrations. It also touches on legal implications of nursing duties. To those already practicing, this book will refresh your knowledge to give your best. To those who are yet to start practicing, it will challenge you to understand that Nursing has to be a calling and not just an opportunity to rush for a job for the sake of the salary it pays. – **Justine Attipoe,** *Dagbamate Health Centre.*

# INTRODUCTION

According to Virginia Henderson, "the unique function of the nurse is to assist the individual, sick or well, in the performance of those activities contributing to health or its recovery (or to a peaceful death) that he (the patient) would perform unaided if he had the necessary strength, will or knowledge." This functional definition of nursing indicates that the individual performing the nursing care; the nurse has a lot of roles to play while empowering the sick or fit individual to regain the necessary will, strength or knowledge to perform unaided.

Most times, it is in carrying out those duties that lots of unfortunate incidences are noticed, some which go ways down to destroy the image of the nurse, the health facility and the image of nursing at large. I admit there are many instances where the definition above has reflected in the cares rendered by most nurses to those who need them. The quality work usually goes unnoticed and unrewarded, but the appalling side receives apprehension. Negligence is quickly noticed than hard work and hence, any little break in a good nature of the nurse's job description may rapidly attract media attentions and exaggerated interactions especially among people who have no or very little knowledge on what nurses do and what nurses are required to do.

For sometimes now, I observed that the nursing profession is losing respect in the eyes of the public and if nothing is done about it, the services of nurses in the future may not be a priority of most individuals. I believe for the sake of the hunger of the media and the rapid growth in the utilization of social media, coupled with the misconception of the general public, amidst lack of trust from families and patients in general, there should be a call for attention and perhaps a colour change in attitude to save the pale image of the career nursing. It is a high time we nurses rise up and work hard to redeem the image of the noble profession; else, something unexpected may overtake us at a stride.

The public image of nursing is important and can never be over looked or taken for granted. When the public image is welcoming, the practice is interesting and there is a great co-operation of the individuals who need the services of nurses. The image people carry in their minds about nurses sometimes is appealing and other times, is appalling. This simply explains that everyone may describe the nurse in general by using the personal experiences they had from their respective encounters with certain practitioners of the noble profession. In this case, I may say the image of the nurse is created by the nurse. In other words, the public opinion of who a nurse is actually, is crafted and shaped by the nurse herself. The nurse has in her hands the tool to shape or destroy the image of her profession. When the nurse is hard working, the public has a positive perception about nurses and vice versa. The image of the nurse hence is to a large extent, is in the hands of the nurse.

In other instances, the effort of the nurse does not matter and does not play any role in the creation or maintenance of reputation whatsoever. The image of the nurse to some extent, in these cases is not in the hands of the nurse. For instance, there are some people who are never satisfied no matter how excellent the care you give them measures. Try your best, die for them, kill yourself for them; they won't be satisfied. There are other people who as a result of jealousy and enviousness for nurses would never like to say anything good about them. I have met few friends who have not been successful at completing nursing schools and had to change their academic courses to pursue something else for certain reasons. I intentionally assessed their conceptions respectively about nursing and I realized they have no good images in mind. Maybe their mistrust is as a result of the anger arising from the incidences of them being rusticated from the nursing schools. To these kinds of people, no matter how hard the nurse works, they are never satisfied and would never appreciate the nurse for a work done because of what has been coded in their minds.

Maybe we have to focus on the former; people whose mental images about nurses are created by the nurses themselves. And let's forget about people who are not appreciative and won't recognize the job of someone dying to save their lives with professional knowledge acquired through studying and practicing. Our job should not be to please people; but to do the right things and whoever perceives the right thing to be inadequate, let his conscience judge him.

This book, simple known as "Noble Letters' contains noble epistles written by a concerned nurse, reminding, informing, encouraging and rebuking nurses and nursing students to change, to improve and inculcate behaviours that would save the sinking image of the nursing practice in all parts of the world, Africa precisely and Ghana most especially. The book serves as a razor to shape the attitude of student nurses and student midwives as they prepare for their career in the future. The goal of the author is to inspire, motivate, educate and remind the nurse to make realistic choice bothering on her communicative and relationship skills, lifestyle, practice and attitude.

In this book the pronoun "she" has been used predominantly to refer to the nurse where it is necessary. "He" was used to represent the patient receiving care from "her". You are informed that as far as nursing is concerned, the nurse can be a "he" or a "she" and so can a patient be. The book has made the above provision in order to directly convey its messages in a simple language. Take note of this and enjoy reading the noble letters.

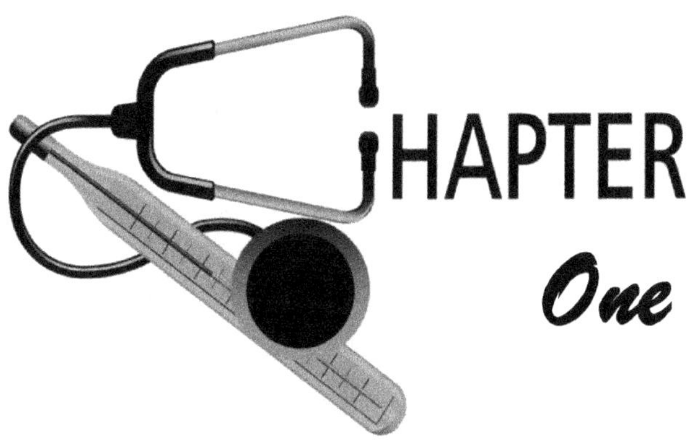

CHAPTER
One


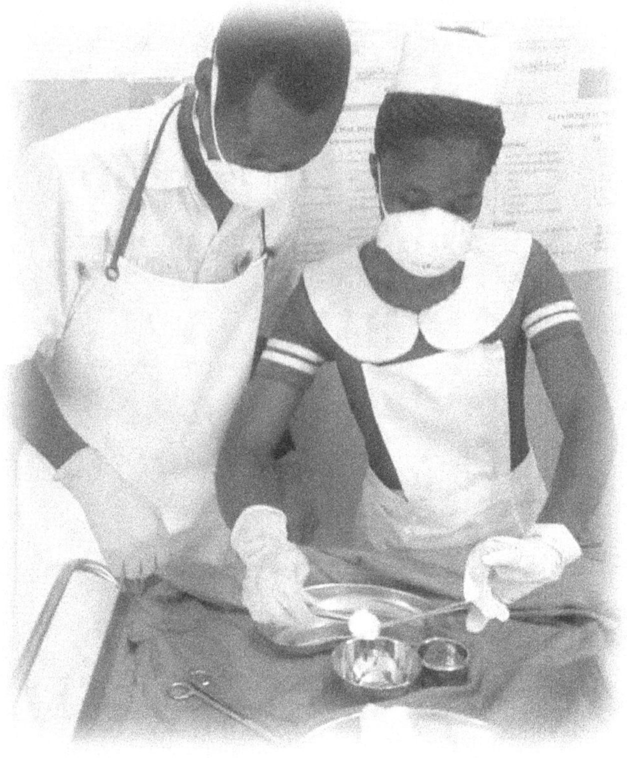

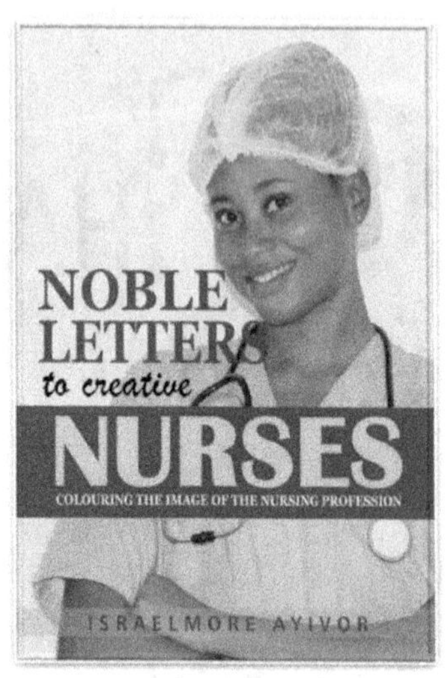


# SOMETIMES YOU WILL NOT HEAR "THANK YOU".

*A letter from,
The Never-Regretting Nurse*

## <u>Nurse, you're my pillow!</u>

*Oh my nurse, please wipe your sweat*
*Never be sad anytime, my bed I wet*
*It is not my will to make you tired*
*Forgive me please, never get me fired*

*Attend to me whenever I call for help*
*It is my pains that make me yelp*
*But I know you understand, my dear angel*
*With your special care, I shall become stable*

*You deserve the honour you don't receive*
*Never look on this and start to grieve*
*Though I have nothing in my pocket to give*
*You said, "I am satisfied when my goals I achieve"*

*You may not hear so many thank you's at all*
*On your inner motivation, stand tall*
*And don't think in vain you suffer and toil*
*You shall be greased with God's own oil*

*You definitely have a double heart, I guess*
*Your work is built on love, I must confess*
*You are always my number one hero*
*On you I rest my head like a pillow*

Israelmore Ayivor

*Dear Nurse,*

Don't forget. Prepare your mind for the worse. Don't always expect compliments from others. If you expect it and it doesn't come, you may become frustrated. But if you don't expect it and it comes, you will be excited. It is not about the compliment; it is about your commitment. What inspires the nurse is likely to be the 90% of her inwardly-built compassion and 10% of her outward-earned compliments. You can do it without a "thank you".

---

One of the usual sources of frustration for nurses is the unappreciative attitude of the people whose lives they hit their heads on rocks to save out of death or complications. I settled on this fact after going through an experience and I also discovered that this issue is all over the place messing up with the art and science of caring, thereby weakening the hard-built pillars of the noble profession. When I did a little survey, I discovered that some people somewhere also experience what I experienced. It's a global matter and hence, it attracted the attention of the never-regretting nurse, the writer. Without delay, he refilled his sacred pen with black ink voluminously, in order to register his concern with an agitated seriousness.

One particular afternoon, I happened to nurse a married woman who was accompanied into my ward by a gentleman she introduced to us as her husband. She complained of lower abdominal pains and all other accompanying signs should inform the emergency nurse to request for pregnancy test. Well, with the recommendation of the doctor, I requested for it with the only woman being aware. Her husband was so caring and was ready to give any support needed by the nurses, yet I never let him know I was requesting for a pregnancy test for his wife to help the nurses and doctors understand her situation better.

The result was ready! It was positive, an interpretation indicating she was pregnant at that moment. I was excited and was about to break the news to the woman, thinking it was going to be a good news to her. I was preparing in my mind to educate her on precautions to take and keep her unborn baby safe. However, I paused to excuse her husband with the intention of telling her alone so that she in turn informs her husband in a romantic way. Under the influence of a Nollywood movie I watched not long ago, I was of the view that the excitement of her husband would be richer if his partner says it, than when the nurse discloses it. I took confident steps and gave a confident smile with a confident wave while extending my hands to the recovering woman; "Hi dear, the result is positive. You are pregnant. Congratulations!", I whispered. "Fuck you! Stupid boy! Get away from me! Stop that lie! I am not pregnant. You are such a naughty being. Leave my bedside now; I said get lost!", she retorted not as someone in pain, but as someone daring an opponent in the boxing ring. She spoke to me with her strong muscles and I couldn't believe what my ears were hearing.

I became sad, very sad because I initially thought I would be greeted with a smile. Thanks be to God, I excused her husband. Well, when hours slipped over hours, she called me close to her bedside, apologized for her thunder-fashioned response and made a passionate request. With her tender lips trembling in rigor, she begged me never to disclose the outcome of her laboratory investigation to her husband. She never wanted him to know she's pregnant. "Why?", I asked. "He just arrived from oversea three days ago. We have not had sex for the past 6 six months since he travelled. I know the man responsible for that result you were interpreting to me. My husband is not the one. When he gets to know it, I will be in trouble the rest of my life." With a sigh, I felt what she felt and reassure her that "God is in control."

The patient's charter tells me every day that the patient has the right to confidentiality. I salute you "Mr. Charter"! The secret remained a secret as she promised to handle it through her biological father. Afterall, my business is to care since caring is the heart of nursing. God being so good, the 2$^{nd}$ World War has ended and I do not want to begin the 3$^{rd}$ World War in someone's house. With my mouth zipped, I carried my two tiny legs, back to my job, caring!

That's a typical example of many instances where nurses are greeted with displeasure after their professional struggles, breaking through rocks, and mountains to save savable lives and to put smile on the faces of people who may not believe there is hope in life again. Sometimes, you think what you are doing is going to make your client appreciative, but it rather turns to make him use acidic and corrosive words on you; I want to believe you have had such an experience before if you're a nurse.

Nurses are also human beings and they also have emotions; in facts multiples of them. Under the conditions they work, the writer of this letter observed that they even have the greater exposure to physical and psychological stress. Nurses go through chains of pains with crafted and gifted hands to help rewrite and lengthen the biographies of people under their care. They do so in hard ways that are risky to even shorten their own biographies. It is like embarking on an adventure to reduce your lifespan by cutting pieces of it and fixing it on the lifespan of another person prolonging his own, and after doing all that, it is not noticed. However, I believe the tough training received by nurses was deliberately schemed to help them stand all these challenges, making them not to be too hungry to receive "thank you".

The frustration of the nurse is not only as a result of the attitude of patients and patient's family members. Other factors are also responsible; some can be manipulated, but others cannot. I think if the source of frustration cannot be adjusted, the nurse herself must rather adjust to go through without trapping harmful pathogens that may infect her inner joy. Some of the causes I picked after doing a little survey among colleague nurses I list as follows;

**Tension from some Physicians:** Sometimes, some doctors seem to multiply the rate of emotional imbalance for nurses by putting them in undue states of anxiety. Commanding, humiliating and condemning seem to be the triggers. Let me not go far with that. Permit me to save my ink by not writing long paragraphs on this.

**Nature of the work**: A nurse may become frustrated after realizing that there is nothing to do to make a patient recover. There is so much stress in handling patients under palliative care. Sometimes, I feel like I should enter the patient's heart or lung and fix something which went wrong.  I become sad when I realize I can't do that.

**Feelings of regret:** This happens when all your efforts to save a life did not work. You may become frustrated; feeling like your effort is wasted. One day, I spent 2 hours with my patient together with other nurses and a doctor to make him recover. It didn't happen as we expected. Though all precautions were taken, I bruised myself on my way to pick up the oxygen cylinder and running up and down cracked me like a broken baobab pod. When he breathed his last breathe, I was almost mad!

**Attitude of governments**: Maybe he doesn't have to write much about this, but to highlight the truth, sometimes, the payment nurses receive is enough to add fertilizer to the frustrations they go through. I might say, the frustrations are originally minor, but the remuneration from "some" government makes the nurses to "major in frustrations". I know young nurses are not like some other professionals who have sky-wide scale of opportunities to earn free fuels and transport mechanisms to facilitate their work. Maybe it happens elsewhere behind the oceans, but kindly remind me if you have seen or heard this good thing happening here. I know some nurses who spend almost all their salaries on their transportation fees to their various work places. So tell me, if she comes to work hungry, do you expect her to smile by magic? Or do you want her to be cheerful by charm? It is a hard-to-swallow truth though, but let us leave it there! I don't want to go far.

The Never-regretting Nurse came across a research conducted by Sharon C. Bolton on *"Changing faces; nurses as emotional jugglers"* in the year 2001 which stressed that Nursing is an emotional work. The outputs of this professional research work highlight the essence of nurses managing emotions during varying times and procedures at their work settings. Emotions can go a long way to affect how you perceive life, having been exposed to peculiar treatment over a long period of time. It is an unfortunate thing to see the work of nurses leading them into negative consequences of emotional risks. That is why it is necessary for the nurse to be guided and reminded, retrained and equipped to handle emotional issues arising before they grow horns or wings. The writer is recommending that the nurse subjects herself to learning and applying knowledge obtained on some of these subjects for her own good. Perhaps she needs to attend personal development conferences, trainings and read books that teach how to handle social, emotional, and occupational issues in order to build herself up over time.

The nurse indeed is prone to emotional juggling; one minute she's smiling, the next minute, she's polite. Then sooner, she becomes sad, and not long she's running into boring times. She would be calm now and the next moment you see her, she's active, if not humorous; or passive if not remorseful. By the time she finishes a shift, she would have hovered around many moods, and swinging from one more to another while on her way home after work. The maintenance of the image of nursing goes at the snail's pace as a result of some of these factors. Until we take the bull by its horn, and just decide to do the hard work without expecting equal rewards, we may never get there sooner.

Sometimes when people blame nurses for what they do, or what they are not able to do, I refer them to what they go through. I heard the attitude of the nurse being painted blacker than that of the devil's cloak and it became the talk of the town and I feel sad for the professionals who have many legal concerns starring them in the face while they boil their blood to cook healing for others to enjoy. I don't feel sad because I am a nurse, and also not because I want to be on the defensive side. But truth be told, until you know the situation a person goes through, you don't blame him for his behaviour in vain. And if you don't know what nurses go through, I am very sorry; all you have to do is to be patient and not say something that would discourage them. You either close your mouth and say nothing, or open your ears and learn something you don't know.

I made a suggestion somewhere concerning this. I watched a nurse who was abused with words by a certain patient's family member. The nurse controlled herself and forced her tears back into her tear glands; refusing every opportunity to shed them. Few minutes after the incidence, a family member of another patient who wasn't aware of any earlier verbal abuse walked in. He greeted the sad nurse with smiles and expected smiles back. Unfortunately, he couldn't receive what he expected from the emotionally stirred nurse and that made him furious. He expressed his fury with insults and this nurse could no longer handle the weight of both abuses happening within 30 minutes. It was like a heavy downpour; no matter how hard you try, you'll get wet when you walk through. She ruptured into an uncontrollable moment of crying. Her eyes, like a broken bottle…draining flood. Her cheek… like a waterfall, full of tears in motions.

My advice is very simple; sometimes, you will never receive "thank you" even if you give the best care. Your motivation should come from within. Nail it on to your mind and never let it fly off. It will help you tomorrow if not today; it helped me yesterday and it's helping me always.

Some patients and their family members underrate the prowess of the nurse even before they set off from the house to a health facility. It is our duty as nurses to convince them beyond every reasonable doubt that we are not just there as "mere workers". We make great contributions. Yes we do. I remember a day when a patient's father asked me a very simple question about his daughter's condition. Just when I was about to answer him, her daughter said, "don't ask him. Ask the doctor. He is just a nurse". "Just a nurse?" Oh no! However, I gave my simple explanation to both and I was fully convinced they were just partially convinced because they still think I am "just" a nurse. When the doctor arrived later, they asked the same question and the doctor gave the same answer I gave.

My patient was sorry and vowed not to underrate the
knowledge of nurses. Yes! Many clients out there think our
main job is to carry the orders of doctors. Wherever you
are, prove them wrong. Let them know we are not just there
for that role.

And now to the creative nurse;

Congratulations on your hard work. You are so strong and
brave, hard to maintain your work ethics in the midst of
downpours of abuse, stress, frustrations and the likes. I may
not see the work you do, but I trust they were built out of
love. This is because it could only take love for you to dare
and handle people with highly contagious diseases, even at
the time you are receiving little or no appreciation. More
grease to your elbows and more health to your bones.
Remember, sometimes you don't receive "thank you" for
the tireless work you are doing. Instead of appreciation,
sometimes it is abuse; abuse from the very people you are
helping; abuse from the very people you are assisting. It is
a difficult thing to handle, but I know, as long as you make
your mind that "sometimes, I may not receive thank you",
you will be fine, happy, smiley, humorous, joyful and
exceptional thankful to yourself because the work you do
serves as the best thank you to you.

You will not regret being a nurse if your mind travels in the
clouds of commitment. When the atmosphere is hazy with
smokes of ungratefulness from the very people you are
contributing to help, be silent and let the clouds of
commitment drop its showers bit by bit and clean the dusts
on the louvers of your expectations. Dear nurse, give all

you can to your patients even if you don't receive droplets of "thank you" in your palms to grease your tired elbows. Wear the gloves of commitment and not with goggles of hunger for appreciation. You will be happy and never regretful.

The image of nursing care is very essential to the state and future of the profession. I understand you may not receive appreciation for whatever you do. But never let it reduce your efficiency and devotion. Never reduce your knowledge and skills to match the remuneration you receive. Never lower your care because of the poor feedback that comes from the very people who receive it. Keep your knowledge at a high professional level and give the best standard of care and together, we shall snatch nursing from the fangs of bad reputation. I trust you will treat my letter with diligence.

This is your friend,
*The Never-Regretting Nurse.*

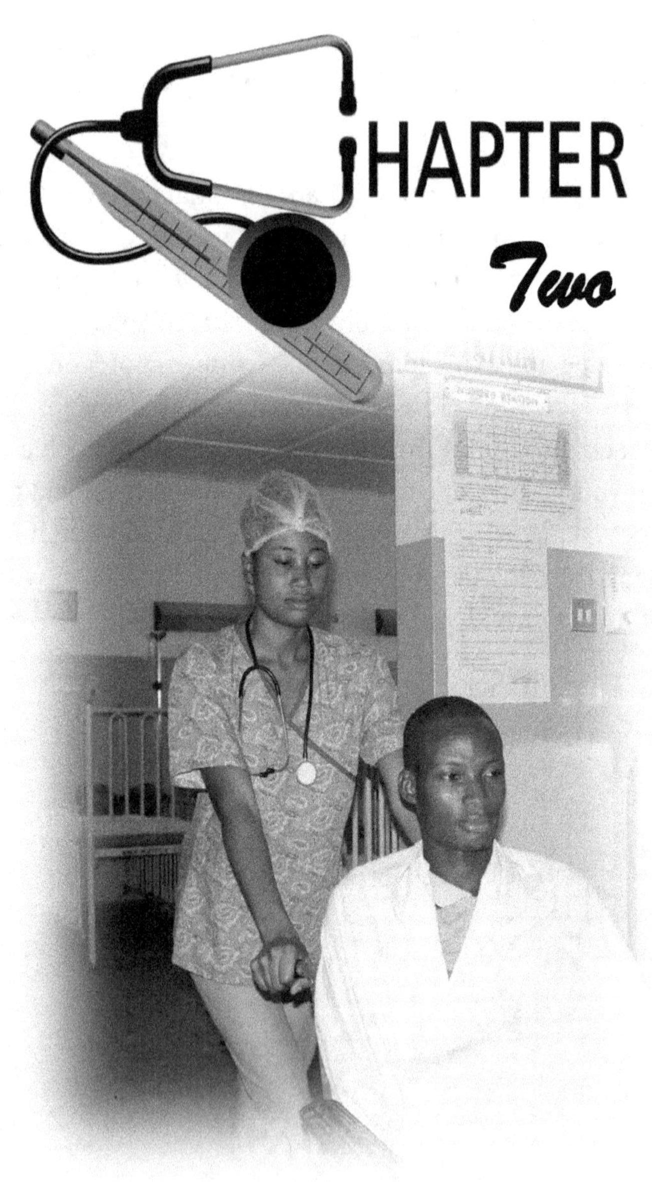


CHAPTER
Two

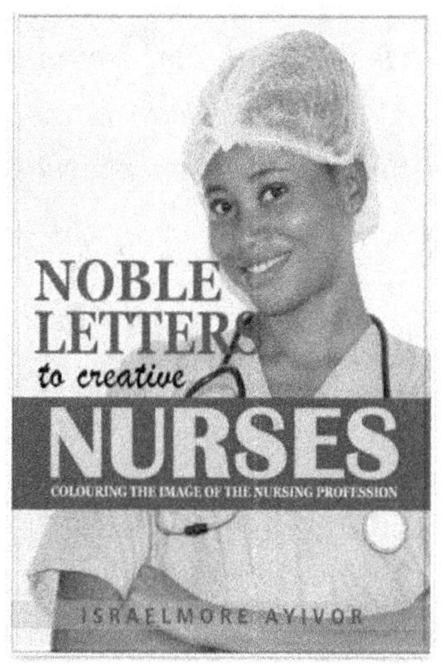

# CARING IS THE HEART OF NURSING

*A letter from,*
*The Care Advocate*

<u>**Help me thank the creative nurse….**</u>

*The polite words of the creative nurse*
*Is richer than the money I have in my purse*
*She advocates for the sick and the weak*
*She does this every weekend and every week*

*Her smiles alone carry a precious balm*
*To grease the joints which suffer harm*
*She did her best to lessen my pain*
*This she vowed to do again and again*

*The dead, I would have been among*
*But look, I'm fine, looking healthy and young*
*Help me thank the tireless nurse*
*Else, my sickness would have become worse*

*Dressed with pride, appearing so smart*
*I believe what she does is from her heart*
*"You will be fine again", she always said*
*Her laughter and smile, I see did not fade*

*Thank you my angel; angel with a stethoscope*
*With your care, the sick sooner or later  can cope*
*You guarded my bedside when I was asleep*
*The fruits of your labour you shall reap!*

Israelmore Ayivor

*Dear Nurse,*

Remember this. If what you do in the ward; from walking to running, to writing, to talking is not contributing towards caring for the patient, you aren't doing it right! Caring is the heart of nursing. When the heart is dead, the entire body stops functioning. In the absence of caring, nursing in itself is sick.

---

In a book written by Toni Morrison entitled "Beloved", lies a simple sentence on a loaded page. It reads; ***"the pieces that I am, she gathered them and gave them back to me in all the right order."*** Though his book isn't about Nursing, the sentence paints a picture of someone whose goal was met. That person was caring and her care mended the broken pieces of another. I don't forget what one of our tutors said to us when I was in the Nursing School. His words, "the most hardworking nurse is found at the dirtiest part of the ward" is real and true and I trust you know this. I understand it deeper when I began to practice and I discovered there is a great difference between knowing something and practicing it. The most hardworking nurse indeed is not the one who runs away from mess patients make. She is found always at the part of the ward where work has accumulated and she makes sure it is well done.

Congratulations to the hardworking nurses. I am mindful they have a "double heart"; one for pumping blood through their own blood vessels and the other for showing concern where and when it's needed. Do you know that "spirit" which can make a caregiver smile sincerely while cleaning the mess caused by the patient? What could inspire the nurse to kick away her "sleep" in order to ensure that the patients under her care are safe, strong, sound and secured? Again, what could make the caretaker starve herself in order to make her patients get satisfied? What is that substance that could make a caregiver forget her pleasure and dedicate her life to securing another person's own?

The last time I watched something weird happened in this life, it was an event of a nurse cleaning the mess of a "mental" patient who soiled himself with a very awfully offensive watery stool in copious volume. Unexpectedly, this patient led by his own feelings spitted a very offensive and thick volume of saliva and it fell right on the cheek of the nurse while she was cleaning his mess. As if her heart was wrapped in layered bundles of empathy, she just smiled, wiped off the saliva which drained down to almost touch her lip. She went on with the cleaning duty as if nothing had happened. She even thanked the uncooperative patient humbly after cleaning him. So what could make a nurse lay his life down for another person to get his life lifted up?

When I found the fitting answers to this repeated question, I picked up the pen to write it down and mail them to anyone who cares. And any nurse who cares I call "The Creative Nurse". The pillar of love is what supports the essence of nursing. In the absence of love, nursing becomes a tough job to handle. In the absence of love, you would see the nurse getting fed up, complaining and getting offended because of loads of messy work that appear to keep increasing each and every hour. When the spirit of love is in you, you will choose to care for someone who needs your skills to survive even when the person is not appreciative. When I was a patient, I experienced the hard work of a nursing student, Grisilder in 2007 at the time I was not yet a nurse, these were the words I wrote about her; "The nurse can make many shinning starts out of a broken moon. Through her, life goes on brightening again even in multiple folds." Kudos to hardworking nurses!

The word "nurse" was derived from the 1550's Middle English word "nurshen" meaning "to suckle a baby", the Latin word "nutricia", meaning "to nurture or to feed" and the Old French word "norture" which means "suckling or nourishment." Before we can actually know the "spirit" that can keep the nurse going, we have to deeply understand the above definition. The definition equates the nurse to a mother who feeds her child. Unless a mother is abnormal, I don't think there is something else that would prevent her from suckling her baby when that baby is hungry. The baby cannot feed himself; he doesn't have a breast. He needs another person to help him do it. The person who feeds him shouldn't get fed up even if the baby urinates on her.

And so in my simple words, I see Nursing as the practice involving contributing toward the health needs of someone who may not know or have the ability to solve that health need. It is only the person who cares that would give out the breast milk she has and let a baby suck it till he is satisfied. That is typically the work of the nurse. She gives out herself so the patient's health can be restored. This lavish attitude can only be dispensed over the counter of love. Love is the mother of caring! My Primary school science teacher taught me that "the heart is the battery of the human body". If it is true, then my suggestion is just simple; right before you dress up from home and set off to work, "charge" your heart with the attitude of caring. It should be fully charged so it won't run down while you are on duty. You will enjoy your practice like never before!

Between the years 1975 and 1979, Dr. Jean Watson, a renowned nursing theorist developed a nursing theory she named "Philosophy and theory of Transpersonal Caring" which has been a helpful contribution to the professional knowledge of the nursing career. In her theory, she explained how nurses care for patients and how the care given transcribes into health promotion and restoration. You may have read about her scholarly work and if you did, this is an opportunity for you to be inspired again. Her theory and other theories of nursing teach us to understand that nursing cannot be practiced without compassion. Compassion is what it takes for you to feel what the patient feels and that would create the willingness for you to work hard to ensure that what makes the patient feels that way is removed so he can be well again.

I mounted my letter on the seven pillars of this theory. And if you care to know the seven assumptions of Dr. Jean Watson's theory, they are as follows, further explained;

**1.. "Caring can be effectively demonstrated and practiced only interpersonally."**

You don't care for someone in your mind. He does not even see what's running in your mind. His body would not respond to what you think about him, but what you do to him. The word "caring" is a practical word.

**2. Caring consists of "carative" factors that result in the satisfaction of certain human needs.**

When you care about someone, that care should lead to a positive outcome. If you pour "urine" into the engine of a car that needs diesel, your intervention is not "carative". Your actions must be helpful if you care.

**3. Effective caring promotes health and individual or family growth.**

There is a degree of improvement in the person you care for. Caring leaves an indelible mark when done free-heartedly and effectively.

**4. Caring responses accept person not only as he or she is now but as what he or she may become.**

Caring is done to achieve a certain goal. When you are doing it, you want to be sure you are on track to get that goal achieved.

**5. A caring environment is one that offers the development of potential whilst allowing the person to choose the best action for him or herself at any given point in time.**

There are many ways to do certain things. When caring for someone, you make use of the best possible step. It's all about going for the best options.

## 6. A science of caring is complementary to the science of curing.

You can't cure if you don't care. When curing becomes your goal without caring, the patient will not even welcome your style of practicing.

## 7. The practice of caring is central to nursing.

Nursing leans on the art of caring. When "caring" falls, nursing cannot stand. Without caring, nursing will become unstable.

Now, since the art of caring is central to nursing, I want to believe that the major role a nurse can play in making her practice helpful is to ensure that everything she does brings hope to the patient and not to rather kill the little hope existing in him initially. Words are like rainbows; they fade quickly; but actions are like the sky; always there as a reminder. Every little action you take on a conscious patient, just assume he is noticing it. And in this letter, I want to remind you, this assumption is always true.

I was assessing the knowledge and beliefs of my patients recently to take note of their expectations as to what the term "caring" means. I discovered that things that make them satisfied aren't things hard to come by. "A nurse who cares is the person who is ready to listen to your complaints even when she is busy. Even if she won't offer a solution, she should just listen to me", a patient told me. Another patient also observed that "a care does not necessarily have to make him feel comfortable now, but it will do so later." These were the word of a patient who felt pains when his wounds were dressed. He knows the art of caring to him is painful initially, but helpful later on. I am charged to accept that obvious fact that there seems to be no compelling, counteracting and controversial reason, thought and idea to argue the statement that "nursing can't be satisfactory without caring."

Caring is the first step towards curing. If you don't care, your method of curing is not complete. It takes caring attitudes to convince a patient to swallow a pill he hates to put in his mouth. Your encouragement, motivation, assurance and reassurance are what it takes to gain your patient's cooperation for your interventions to be appropriate. I know you know; I am just writing to remind; to remind you that when you do more of the good you are already doing, it becomes better. And there are available evidences to justify the fact that when you do more of what you do better, it becomes the best. A nursing order which is lacking an aspect of caring is not worth be utilized for intervention. There is a high chance and I take a middle-ground position to argue out loud that it will not result in achieving a SMART goal or objective criteria.

By the time you are dressing up to go to work, the air surrounding your ears should start reminding you that you are on the journey to care about someone else. The issue of whether to develop a caring attitude or not is not an option as far as nursing is involved; it is a priority. I don't mean to say you are less important when it's time for caring for another person, but that is what I see most hardworking nurses do. They keep their own comforts under detention in order to ensure that their patients' comforts become evident. In some cases, you see nurses tired, but willing to stretch and do more.

When I was a nursing student, I worked with a midwife who was pregnant and was in pain while assisting in the delivery of another woman in labour. She had no one to complain to concerning her pains at that moment. She endured it and made sure the other baby was delivered safely before seeking attention for hers. Her own pain could not limit her work. Given the centrality of this issue, this is what nurses and midwives do. An outsider of the nursing family may stand in one dark corner somewhere and say things they want to say. They must not be given a lion-portion of blames for what they say because perhaps they have termite-size knowledge on what nurses go through to make the nursing process successful.

And now to the creative nurse; congratulations to you for your determination to offer your care kindly to those who need it. You are creating many bright starts from broken moons though no one, or only few people seem to recognize it. If it hadn't been through you, pain wouldn't have been elevated and not alleviated. Do your job wholeheartedly, smiling from ear to ear and grinning from cheek to cheek. Paint a beautiful colour of hospitality, empathy and selflessness using permanent markers on the precious chambers of your heart. I may not have notes and coins of different currencies to spread on your head as a sign of appreciation. But simply, I say you are doing an amazing job. I charge you to do more for God and for mankind.

As long as you are eager to see someone healed, may you be strengthen to make it happen. Since a weak person cannot do much, may God sustain and increase your strength to become the strength to the weak. But please and please, when you see a nurse who is lacking the qualities you have, fold this letter in a gentle way and give it to her. Tell her it is unfortunate I am too far and may not reach her because of my distance, so I pen down something she would be glad to read. Remind her to pause and think through her old decisions and encourage her to start doing "dusting" to clean the dirty corners of her attitude. Tell her to sniff the joy of caring through her nostrils. I am mindful that when she do this, she would breath with relief and enjoy the ventilation of the inner benefits of caring. Let her remember that caring is about

- Becoming sensitive to the needs of others.
- Giving the support others need from you.
- Instilling hope in the hopeless.

"Maybe this one moment, with this one person, is the very reason we're here on earth at this time", said Jean Watson, the nursing theorist. Since iron sharpens iron, one human being is needed to make another human being stronger. Be that caregiver. I trust that your tiny but faithful contributions will add to the little but honest contributions of others and together we shall build a clear and clean ocean of nursing reputation with droplets of many caring activities, where the world will find a source to quench it's thirst for good health, and solace to swim safely in the mighty name of Nursing care.

Do enjoy your morning, afternoon and night duties!

Sincerely yours,
*The Care Advocate.*

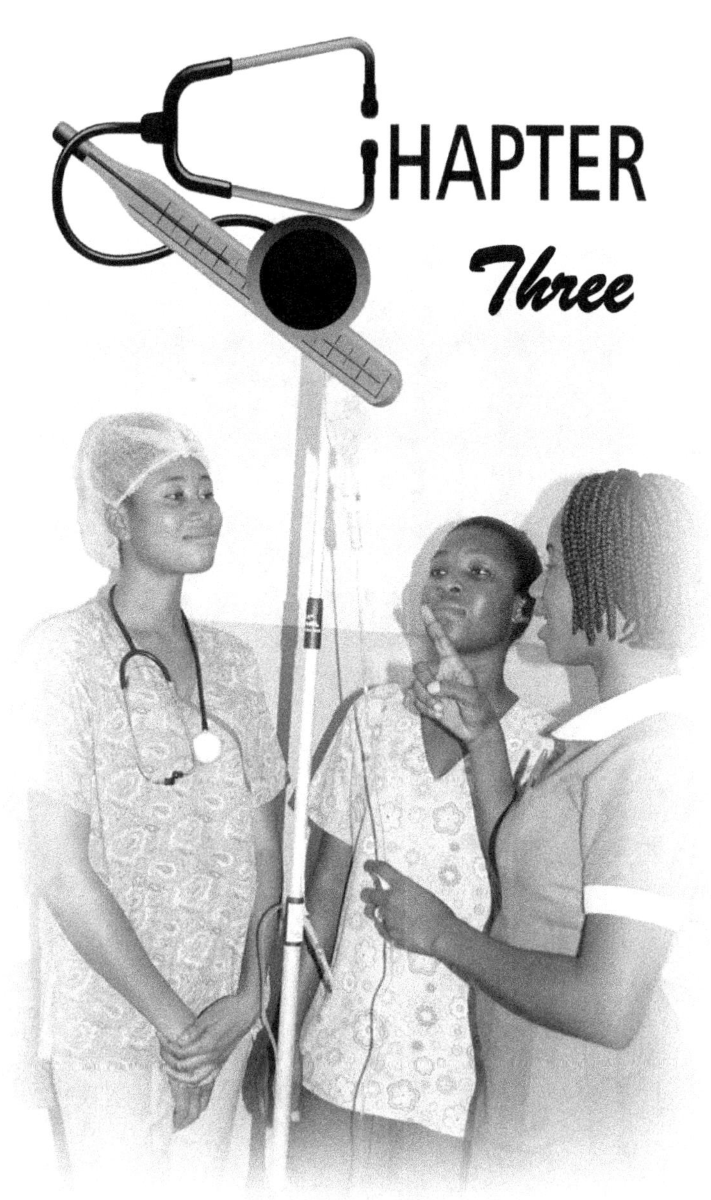

# CHAPTER Three

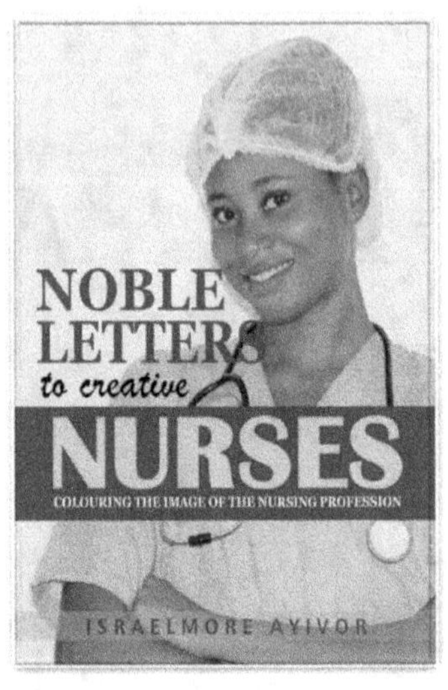

# ORNAMENTS OF THE NURSING PROFESSIONS

## A letter from

## The Nurse "Beautician"

<u>**The beauty of nursing is in your hands**</u>

*The beauty of nurses is in their characters*
*How they speak to patients; it really matters*
*You decide to make nursing appealing*
*If your choice of words is not appalling*

*The beauty of the nurse is in her care*
*Her care is special, honest loving and fair*
*You decide to make nursing attractive*
*If your words and actions are not repulsive*

*The beauty of the nurse is in her compassion*
*The patient's recovery is her main intention*
*You decide to make nursing beautiful*
*If your care is exceptionally wonderful*

*The beauty of the nurse is in her attention*
*That alone to the patient is a deep inspiration*
*You decide to make nursing praiseworthy*
*If your relation with the patient is trustworthy*

*The beauty of a nurse is in her energy and power*
*With which she cares for the sick every hour*
*You decide to make nursing a noble career*
*If you offer your best even against every barrier*

---

Israelmore Ayivor

*Dear Nurse,*

Your reminder; Nursing is beautiful; don't fade it. Ensure you colour it with the best attitude and you will make the profession stand nobler among her sister professions. You have the pool of tools in your hands; don't use them to scratch and disfigure the face of your career. Rather use them to shape it. The better the attitude of the nurse, the more attractive Nursing becomes to those who need the nurses' services. I know you can; God knows you will. Make it happen.

---

S orry to disappoint you this time. This letter doesn't contain anything new. If you want to see and read something new here, you have missed the target. The letter from the Nurse-Beautician is just a reminder to you. Old rules made new; old principles re-polished; the same things you already know as a nurse are the same things you are going to be reminded of here. The exception to this rule is the student nurses whose interest is beaming up desirously with hopes that one day they will find themselves in the shoes of professionals. They would find this piece, perhaps as new as a day old chick. Keep this letter in a safe file and when new daughters and sons are born in our profession, use the words in it to baptize them.

Not long ago, something big fell on my head and kept me scratching my sculp. I beg to announce it. It is the definition of the word "principle". I have read close to 41 definitions of the word "principle" from about 32 different websites and blogs. I came across tens of phrases in which the word "principle" was used and almost a hundred of sentences in which it is found. I'm already done with 6 books that defined the word; however, none of those definitions were so satisfactory to me than the one I found at vocabulary.com. It came in just 13 words and simply reads, "a principle is a kind of rule, belief or idea that guides you." Briefly, I learnt from this simple but discerning definition that a principle is a mechanism through which an objective is achieved. It means you may dream big about an objective; you may make millions of plans to make it happen, but if you don't use the principles that should lead you to the success you chase, you are toiling in vain.

To make it clearer, kindly permit me to use the automobile principle to explain the concept I am building up here. The builder of the car tells us that this car must operate with "petrol". It means without petrol, the car will not move; and it also means with petrol, it will move. That is a principle! You may be the finest prince on earth, you may be the cutest queen alive; if you disobey that principle, the car won't move. Maybe you decided to pour urine into the car's engine in place of the diesel; maybe you think palm nut soup will do the job. You can even add white porridge or coca cola drink if you like. Or try orange or pineapple juice and see it for yourself. Until you bring in the petrol, this car will never move. Principles don't really care about how many square meals you take per day. They are insensitive to your negotiations. They call for rapt obedience. Just obey the principle irrespective of whether you are a Christian or you are a Muslim or whatever. The principle does not consider your age, race, creed or political affiliation. Just obey it.

I see that the standard of nursing is falling as a result of many factors. These factors are quickly succeeding in eating away the fabrics of the principles of nursing practice. One of them is the way and manner in which we drop down our values and no longer appreciate our ethics as we get old at post. The same things apply to student nurses whose strong linens of politeness and courtesy begin to develop perforations as their years in school increases from zero to one, one to two and so by the time they are completing, the humility with which they enter the school on day one doesn't exist anymore. As if they are no longer essential, the rules with which schooling or practicing began, soon becomes forgotten rules. If we want to suture the lacerated reputation of nursing and ride happily with pride for the profession to earn the respect it is losing, we must go back and lift the principles we dropped. We must revisit our ethics and right from there, our standard will receive life again. To those who still keep these rules, I believe you are the people resuscitating the profession in this crucial decade. We shall assist you and bring back to life the dying standard. We shall hoist the flags of pride with bold hands, to campaign against the unprecedented sabotages we ourselves have slapped our profession with and fixed back the wings we pulled out that made our successes difficult to fly high. And when it happens, we ourselves will benefit so much.

Without much ado, I want to share with you the 7 essential things I observe we must go back and pick and make our radical pursuit to re-inculcate in us and in our protégés. When our fever of enthusiasm for change escalates the ordinary, better results in the name of good reputation will creep in our faces and nobody will need to come from far to tell us that we have done a wonderful job. The Nurse-Beautician is not making a new rule though; neither is he I passing a new law. This writer is just giving us a reminder. Perhaps, not all may be forgotten laws to you, but some may have definitely been ceaselessly tempering with your competence as a professional. Maybe the ones you practice are the ones someone defaulted and vice versa. Together we shall make nursing great again. And now, the rules;

**Respect your senior nurses:**

The respect for seniors is almost gone and the older nurses and midwives can testify to this. Their style and manner of respect for their seniors in the past is not what is seen now. If juniors can be submissive, we will see more improvement. However I believe seniors in the profession also have roles to play to induce the spirit of respect in their juniors. Until we fill the dry wells with respect for one another, nursing as a profession may continue to be smitten by sudden spasms related to prolong thirst for a good image.

**Communicate politely:**

You are as beautiful as the way you talk. You may have a good point, but if you convey it rudely, you have scratched the nursing profession with rusted metallic comments to look ugly. Speak politely and use friendly words when communicating with your clients. I have not worked with Nurses and Midwives Council of Ghana, neither have I visited the camp of NCLEX. But let's see one of these their possible examinable multiple choice question;

Question number 24:

"Assuming you are a nurse on duty and a newly admitted, known alcoholic, drunken patient accidently fell off from the bed, which of the following will be appropriate to tell him while lifting him to his bed."?

A. Look, don't come and add your troubles to my troubles this evening.
B. Have you seen how far alcohol has taken you?
C. I am sorry. Are you hurt? Oh sorry, let me lift you to the bed again.
D. I knew it. I knew you won't listen. The next time you fall, you will sleep on the floor.

No human being in his or her right senses, daring to pass a much awaited exam will meet this questions and pick A, B, or D. Even if the candidate is not a nurse, he/she will never pick up A, B, or D. Everyone would thick C and when the result comes, he/she would rejoice and say "I have made it!". You have made what? Wait and let's go into the ward.

Right in the ward, imagine you have worked for 10 hours continuously in a night with blackout, using a lamp and never sitting down even for five minutes. All of a sudden, a fight broke between two patients who were long-time secret rivals at home before they were admitted close to each other. In the fight, both were wounded, giving you another tough work to do! How will you talk when cleaning their wounds respectively? Now, stop imagining and face reality. It is easy to pass exams than to put into practice what made you to pass. Let's leave that there.

When you are polite, one benefit you will gain is that, other people will be careful as to how they talk to you. If you are rude, you are likely to hear people talk to you rudely. Most times, I notice that generally, people who are rude are rather the people who crave for respect and when they don't get it, they become uncontrollably rude. It doesn't work that way. If you think of decorating the world with flowers, begin with a rose seed at your doorstep. Know how to talk good to people and they will respond better.

**Know the names of your clients:**

This is a hard task, but when you begin to practice it several times, you will become a master at it. And bear it in mind that the hardest tasks are always animated by noble pride. It is not the best to call your patient or client "that man", "that woman", "the tall girl", "the ulcer boy", etc. We were taught in school to address patients by their titles, names or whichever nickname they appreciate being called with. When you call a patient by the name he loves, you add concrete value to the therapeutic relationship you are building using the nursing process.

**Never ever discriminate:**

At the nursing school, we were told several times not to underestimate, or discriminate against anyone old or young, poor or rich, literate or illiterate, God-believing or God-doubting. I want to submit to you that the air of discrimination carries more killer pathogens than the sputum of a T.B patient. In the nurse's pledge, you would remember that there is a phrase that frowns on allowing politics, race, creed and religious affiliation of a patient to determine how you show commitment in rendering your duty to him. This is a just a reminder of things you already know. When you bend on underestimating and discriminating patients in your care, you are working hard to reduce the muscle tones of the image of the profession that put food on your table. I know you won't love it when someone discriminates against you. Well, even if you would love it, your patient won't. Let's go for what the patient would want.

**Maintain confidentiality:**

This is among one of the most critically upheld ethics in the nursing profession. I congratulate nurses on this and trust we shall continue to keep it up. Most nurses have exhibited a well-bred mixture of honesty and loyalty when it comes to issues of confidentiality. However, there are few instances that some yet-to-change nurses unintentionally or intentionally end up sharing confidential information to unqualified destinations. You will not know the effects until you get into trouble. Look, this world is already filled with weird events of morbid horrors and you don't want to add a wig or twig of embarrassment to the numberless already on file. I must admit that the major reason why some things are taken for granted is that a few or nobody was held a victim yet. The fact that you have not been caught doing a bad thing does not mean it is the right thing. Let carefulness be my, your and our guide.

**Dress properly:**

Concerning the dressing code of nurses, the least said, the better. I admire nurses in uniform, but I'm also concerned about what nurses do while in the uniform. Let be reminded that the dressing code had two wings. The first has to do with the type, shape, colour, length, neatness and decency of the uniform while the second has to do with the behaviour of the nurse in the uniform. We were taught certain things we must not do when in uniform which my pen won't love to inscribe in this noble epistle. Let's just comply. Dressing code is a tool to boost professionalism. I know there may be some people who would rebuke me that "instead of talking about salary, you're writing about dressing code and uniform". Please, you can do that to me through a private mail, in reply to my letter…"lol"

**Control your emotions:**

With an inexpressible plea of concern, the writer is on his knees. He acknowledges the fact that, you may have your personal weaknesses as a human being. Of course everyone has some. But issues from home that no one else knows nothing about, don't let them run your shift together with you and interfere with your work. I am not sure "anger" is on the duty roster to work with you. Let it go! The patient you nurse is not responsible for that issue you have. The writer, with a high glow of gratitude for your service to mankind is also begging you that as soon as you are about to walk into your facility, hang any anti-nursing issue you have in your heart at the entrance of your facility. When you close from your work, you can pick it up and take it home, provided it is essential to you. But allowing it to follow you, no, no, no, no!

On controlling of emotions, it is my candid suggestion that nursing students be taken through series of teachings that could help them develop themselves in that regard. Microbiology is great, Anatomy is wonderful, but a nurse who has so much knowledge mixed up with bad character won't make her clients enjoy good nursing services. The nursing class is made up of students from various homes and tribes with diverse cultures and lifestyles. We must be careful to prune them to become unbeatably presentable at the field of work. Compulsory, regular and dynamic conferences and training sessions on attitude building, I think can be the way out. Some hospitals do organize in-service trainings to nurses on issues concerning attitude shaping among others and I commend them for that. But with my experience, I am convinced that the very people who need such conferences are the people who absent themselves with so many excuses. Well, let me end it there.

Abdellah Faye, a renowned Nursing theorist, did a fantastic job when she outlined 21 Nursing Problems as part of her postulation in the year 1960. It is a good list of notes she created to help improve our patient-centered approaches to nursing. When I went through the 21 Nursing problems, I discovered she stressed on attitude, emotions, communication, relationship and personal development. About 6 problems out of the 21 were about these aforementioned characteristics and these 6 on the list looking like objectives of a nursing care plan are;

1. To identify and accept positive and negative expressions, feelings, and reactions
2. To identify and accept interrelatedness of emotions and organic illness
3. To facilitate the maintenance of effective verbal and nonverbal communication
4. To promote the development of productive interpersonal relationships
5. To facilitate awareness of self as an individual with varying physical, emotional, and developmental needs
6. To accept the optimum possible goals in the light of limitations, physical and emotional

I am sure that before a nurse can identify emotions of the patient and discover what accounts for them, she must be taught how to manage her own emotions first. The nurse must be taught how "to accept optimum possible goals in the light of limitations, physical and emotional" as Faye postulated. When much is given to the nurse, much can be required of her. Whatever shall contribute towards making the nurse's emotional intelligence rich should be added to her training. Her training should not solely depend on knowledge acquisition on medical and surgical subject areas. Rather, personal management should be intertwined with other science and art related courses to make her a holistic individual, ready to face matters arising in her career. I am grateful to the tutor who taught me "body mechanics". However, as a fan of Oliver Twist, I was to ask for more; "Mental Mechanics" could be added.

On November 4, 2013, Ghana Registered Nurses Association (GRNA) page on Facebook shared a portion of the nurses pledge that reads; "I promise that my personal life shall at all times bring credit to my profession." This simple piece of didactic information received cherished comments from readers, one of which I fell in love with more. In a very noble comment, a reader wrote;

"Personal life includes all aspects of social interaction, religion education, on the job, family, finance, leisure, love and sex life. People know us to be professional nurses whether we are in uniform or not."

She added that "We should not forget the toil our predecessors went through to bring nursing this far. It is left to us young and coming nurses to maintain this integrity or improve upon it and not to tarnish it."

Blending other comments, I want us to get these warning signs that nursing is on the line, shaking to fall and when it fall, posterity shall never forgive us. These I call the 10 anti-nursing factors;

1. When a nurse tells one patient's secret to another person being a nurse, patient or family without the patients approval.

2. When the nurse becomes defensive when someone
   questions her wrong behaviour while she is fully aware
   she was wrong.
3. When you receive gifts from patients and that motivate
   you do work harder than before on or for the giver of
   the gifts.
4. When you talk ill about the competence of other co-
   workers at your workplace to patients or anyone else.
5. When you give an unrealistic promise to the patient or
   relative; a promise you definitely know cannot be
   fulfilled.
6. When you give some patients special attention than
   others and get more affiliated them to the neglect of
   others.
7. When you feel you have a better understanding of the
   patient's problems than anyone else in your ward and
   underrate the contribution of other co-workers.
8. When you unlawfully keep the personal properties
   belonging to the patient in your private custody.
9. When you discredit the profession in front of people
   who already disregard or doubt the competence of
   nurses.
10. When you read the letter of the Nurse-Beautician and
    still do what is not expected and destroy the beautiful
    image of nursing.

When you do the above and the likes of them, you are
distorting the dazzling order of beauty with which nursing
attracted the world in the former days. I am sure you are
much familiar with make-ups that most people use to
enhance the beauty of their outer bodies. The nurse

beautician wishes there could be similar make ups in form of capsules that when swallowed, could enhance the inner beauty of a person. Sadly, there is no such make-up; inner character is not a surface thing, but a deeper lasting bundle of beauty.

When you practice what you have been taught with diligence and hard work, you add an ornamental beauty to the Nursing profession. I know together we shall paint Nursing with strips of beautiful colours. When this happens, others at a distance will be attracted and enjoy our services when necessary. Together, let's make Nursing great again.

And now to the creative nurse; treat this letter with pure hands. When you it gets into your hands, make two copies. Paste one copy on the chambers of your heart and deposit the other into your mind. Be forever reminded that no one can achieve anything by disobeying the principles that requires the expected success to show its unfamiliar face. I am pleased you are doing something right to make someone's health right. You can do better and I know you will. I wrote a sheaf of letters for you to read, keep and share so that together we can enjoy the beauty of nursing not made in China, not made in Japan, but made in you.

Share my greetings with every nurse at your facility. Tell them I may or may not know them, but I love them so much.

Regards upon regards,

*The Nurse-Beautician.*

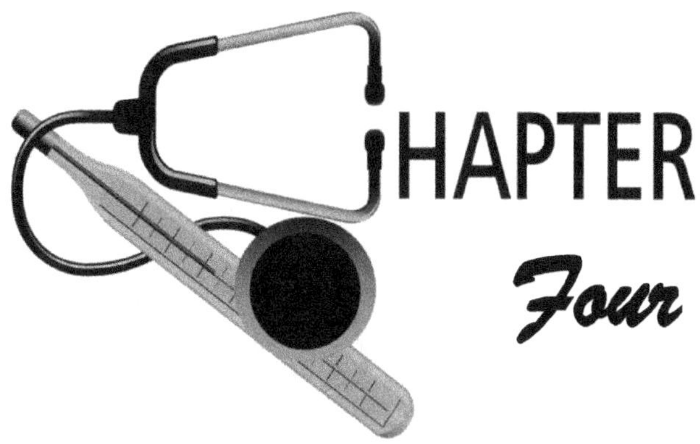

# CHAPTER
## Four

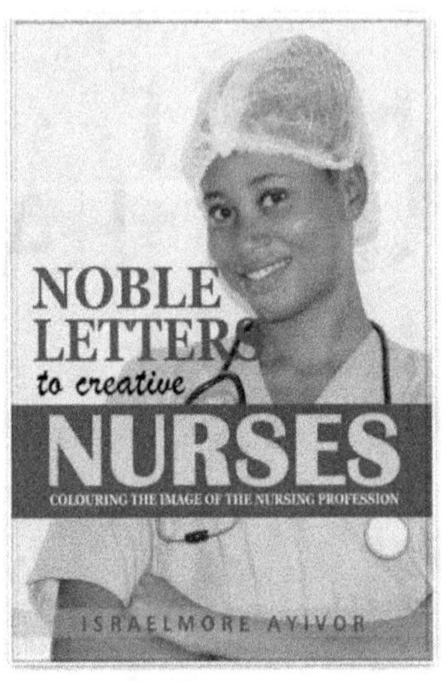

# NURSING IS RELATIONSHIP BUILDING

*A letter from*
*The Nurse-Counselor*

# <u>How I see the creative nurse</u>

*I see creative nurses the way I see divine angels*
*They guard my bed and my room's angles*
*A creative nurse becomes everything to me*
*Until I become stable again and I can be*

*I see the creative nurse the way I see the seamstress*
*Working tirelessly even through her stress*
*She brings my thorn and broken self altogether*
*The pieces she makes perfect when they gather*

*I see creative nurses the way I see mothers*
*About what's happening to me she bothers*
*What I was not able to do, she does for me*
*This is kindness, another mother I see*

*I see the creative nurse the way I see a bus*
*She deserves a clap for her devotion to us*
*She take me from illness to health; she's not cruel*
*She can do it better even without a fuel*

*I see the creative nurse the way I see a brave leader*
*With a care plan to see me climb a healthy ladder*
*She gave right orders to help resolve my conditions*
*And carries them out with thoughtful interventions*

---

Israelmore Ayivor

*Dear Nurse,*

Just to remind you. The success of your nursing goals is dependent on the quality of your relationship with your patient. However, before you can be in good relationship with someone, you must have a good relationship with yourself. A spike of therapeutic rapport, unmingled with personal interests, inordinate affections and jealousy is enough to create an atmosphere of liberty for the definition "Nursing is caring" to be proven again and again.

---

If we are interested in redeeming the fallen image of nursing, a very important corner to start doing our dusting is the nurse-to-patient relationship corner. This is the place where cobwebs leisurely lie and until we consider this, we shall live in the dirt of poor nursing image and keep asking "how?" The success of the nursing management in all parts of the world, Ghana inclusive, falls and rises on relationships. The paradigms of Florence Nightingale's theory of Nursing teach us to understand the essence of relationship between the nurse, her patient and the environment where she nurses the patient. The essence of human to human relationship cannot be underestimated and is mainly essential for the development and maintenance of trust. In the case of nursing, the nurse benefits as a result of gaining the patients cooperation and the patient also derives the benefit of expected recovery. Our relationship skills as nurses when trained at the faculty of professionalism and sandwiched by trust and mutual respect, will put nursing on a reputable page in the world's diary of most respected professions.

Using the nursing care plan, you are expected to achieve your goals within a specified time as indicated in your objective criteria. In the presence of a trustworthy relationship, you can achieve the goals easily. However when trust is missing, your goals will keep hanging because the patient or his family may not give you the needed assistance for you to intervene as required by your orders. Trust is like a bullet. No matter how new the gun is, it is still useless without bullets. That is how nursing and trust are and must lather like soap and water.

According to Mok and Chiu (2004), trusting relationships grossly influence the style of caring by the nurse and in that regard, the nurse who develops the best trusting relationship end up demonstrating the best holistic care, and shows understanding of the patient's social, physiological and physical needs whether they are voiced out or not. Reliability, proficiency and competency of care, hence are founded in the way the nurse relates with the patient.

The relationship of the nurse may vary from day to day depending on the state of the patient. Calnan and Rowe (2005) observed that the relationship of the nurse and the patient is dynamic and alters as long as the care progresses. This was well proven when Hildegard Peplau in her Nursing Theory she called the interpersonal theory outlined four phases of the nurse- patient relationship as;

- Orientation phase
- Identification phase
- Exploitation phase
- Resolution phase

So what happens and what are the roles of the nurse during these four phases of relationship building? The job of the Nurse-Counselor is to discuss them briefly for your reminder in this noble letter.

**Orientation phase:**

The patient comes as a stranger and the nurse defines his problem(s). Once problems are defined, the type of service is decided. The nurse's role at this time includes but not limited to interviewing the patient to come out with the best and most prioritized nursing diagnosis in the next phase, and explain patient's role in assistance with the nurses towards his own recovery.

**Identification phase:**

The nurse picks up appropriate professional roles to work on the patient. The nurse begins to feel the patient belongs to her and that belongingness increases her desire to care for him. It is proven several times that people care for what belongs to them with non-slow-footed passion than what belongs to others. "Owning" the patient during the identification phase adds "adrenaline" to the nurses' commitment. A nurse must be very careful at this stage because the patient might misinterpret her actions as intimate "sympathetic' or "parasympathetic" feelings of love that could lead to deeper relationships.

The expression of interest in the welfare of the patient by a female nurse, coupled with curiosity borne out of the passion to achieve her SMART goals is enough to leave a male patient wondering if this female nurse could make a good wife. It may happen otherwise when the nurse is a male and the patient, a female. This happens mostly when the patient has never received or experienced therapeutic attentions of such nature at home before. There must be clear-cut explanations to drop down unhealthy expectations. The patient is diagnosed during this phase and orders are outlined for intervention in the next phase.

**Exploitation phase:**

There is prioritization of nursing interventions to ensure expected recovery of the patient. The patient's needs, culture, values and interests are taken into consideration. There are more deeper interviews to enable the nurse regulate her care in order not to violate patient's beliefs. When recovery signs begin to appear, the nurse begins to prepare the patient's mind towards the next phase. At the exploitation phase of relationship building, goals could be met fully or partially. Amending care for partially met goals would require deeper interviews. The longer it takes for a goal to be achieved, the longer the exploitation phase lasts.

The identification and exploitation phases may push the nurse into assessment of the patient's body from head to toe. When this is to be done, it should be done professionally so as not to create an atmosphere of offence and low self-esteem for patients. Lack of privacy may collapse your therapeutic walls and physically challenge your relationship to become defective, ineffective or disabled. Be careful how you expose the private parts of the patient since that may lead to unintended consequences.

**Resolution phase:**

There is a professional termination of the relationship at this phase. This happens either because the needs of the patient have been met or further needs of the patient must receive attention in another facility (referral). The patient and the nurse break the bond existing between them and there is a consensus or an emotional balance at the end of the breakage of the bond.

It would not be complete to just inform you on the relationship phases the nurse goes through in giving the needed care without telling you the things to avoid doing in order to stay on track. During the nurse-patient relationship phases, avoid doing the following;

**Condemning the patient when he reveals a bad life history.** For instance, when a patient tells you he is addicted to alcohol, you don't condemn him. That should rather give you an idea on which kind of health education to offer him. You must even be lucky to have a patient who is willing to uncover the naked truth to you. That is a good point to enable you to establish a competent nursing process.

**Interrupting the patient unnecessarily when he is sharing a sensitive matter.** Some patients do forget what they are saying when they are interrupted. Typical examples are dementia patients and those suffering from memory loss. Don't interrupt them quickly. Give them the sky-wide volume of chance to flow. Constant indulgence in frequent interruptions may hide more information you need in order to give the best care.

**Discussing issues outside the problems and needs of patient related to his condition.** You don't go discussing trivial issues that do not contribute to the health needs of the patient. For instance, discussing business, politics, sport and religious issues that could make you deviate from the main purpose of admission should be checked. You may engage patients using diversional therapies and still achieve your nursing goals. However, if there is no need for that, why try it?

**Giving patient unrealistic promises and impossible expectations:** Tell the truth to the patient. Never tell lies in order to make him glad. Supposing you assure a patient that he is going to be fully healed on day 3 of admission, and he still has symptoms on day 5, he may begin to mistrust you the next time you are giving an assurance or reassurance. That is a colossus evidence enough to bring down his trust for you from the sky to the grave. You should assure, but not with unrealistic promises.

**Impersonating; telling patients you are the person that you are not.** I have heard this several times, some nurses (especially trainees) claiming they are doctors. Other times too, orderlies tell patients they are nurses. What will you gain denying your own identity? If you want to create trust, never do that. Stand distinct to correct patients when they misname you. When the patient calls you "doctor", you may respond to him and later remind him that you are a nurse and not a doctor.

As you have read earlier, the nurse must be aware that some patients during the process of caring for them may develop a more intimate interest in them. For instance, there have been several instances where male patients fall in love with female nurses and vice versa. The nurse should be aware that this type of relationship can affect the therapeutic relationship and must be tactical enough to make good judgments. This is a very serious matter and I would love to hit double hammers on it three times daily for thirty days and more. I trust that there is a high possibility of the nurse meeting his/her wife/husband during the course of work. That is possible. However, a professional approach devoid of intimate ideas during the above phases could save nursing reputation. There is more time after the resolution phase for friendship to be born.

Other relationships important in the nursing care include;

**Nurse – Nurse relationship.**

This has to do with how the nurse relates with another nurse in the ward. It is crucial to the nursing process when two or more nurses who are have personal issues against each other are put to run the same shift. You know what I mean. I won't throw more light on this, but I believe in our human ecosystem, there is a wide room for diversity which makes individual values, attitudes, temperaments and characters to differ from person to person. If two nurses cannot lather well upon dialogues and mediations, I don't think there should be need for them to work at the same ward. However, I also think sometimes the causes do not bother on personalities, but rather on personal issues that remain unsolved or become poorly solved. Handling of internal conflict should be a skill every nurse especially nurse managers and ward in-charges must not only know, but also practice and teach. As to whether the nurses will be willing to attend such conferences where these skills are taught, is another thing we should be thinking about.

**Nurse – Employer relationship.**

This has to do with how the employer of the nurse and the nurse mean to each other. To the employer, the nurse is a payee; to the nurse, the employer is a payer. Any disagreement relating to terms and conditions of the service rendered can lead to mistrust and the clients become the sufferers. Imagine nurse who has not been paid goes to work on hungry stomach; how strong is her commitment to work going to be? Meanwhile if she absents herself, using hunger as the excuse, she may be apprehended if not reprimanded. Sometimes too, it is not about payment, but about incentives and conditions under which the nurse works. When the equipment, the know-how staff strength is okay, the nurses will put in more effort. I urge employers; government, quasi or private to address pertinent issues that can drop down the commitment of the health workers when it is at their reach to do. However, if a little opportunity or equipments is made available to the nurse for work, she should never be blamed for not being able to give much.

## Nurse – Other health workers relationship.

The nurse doesn't work on the patient alone. The laboratory technician, the dispensary staffs, orderlies, medical officers, laundry attendants and others in the healthcare team are important to the success of health care. The nurse must hence form a healthy, rocky-founded relationship with all the workers in the health team so as to get a speedy attendance when their services are needed. Sometimes, the attitude of other workers in the health team may not be the best to you. However, your reaction in times of dissatisfaction with the attitude of any staff will determine the outcome of your relationship with them. Here, your choice of words and style of communication is crucial.

And now to the creative nurse,

Dear, I am aware that nobody can have a good relationship with another person without having a good relationship with him/herself. Your expectations about how you love someone else will surprisingly appear darkened in your eyes if your love for yourself doesn't have firm grounds to stand on. You give what you have. If you hate yourself, you can't love others. I urge you to develop a good intrapersonal relationship and settle issues with and within yourself first. Heal yourself of any emotional distress and wipe off any dirt of self-hatred and low self-esteem on the shelves of your conscience. This will help you to love yourself and when you do so, you will love others without a flight of pretense and you will make your relationship with others trustworthy.

The Nurse-counselor is advising that you should never let the features of your non-verbal art of speaking, express a temperamental acrimony of harsh truculence. Endless shifting moods aren't the problem. The problem is when you harbour those moods as a result of embarrassments and deny every opportunity to endeavour and smile away the loads of emotional chagrins. Anytime you talk, pause and ask yourself if your speeches aren't diverting the reputation of nursing into alien gutters.

Strengthen yourself in time of distress and when the need arise; get helped by people who can help you do it. A weak person cannot lift another weak person; they will both break the door of comfort and end up sharing unutterable sorrows in equal proportions. Your strength is important to help recover the lost strength of your clients. The image of nursing cannot be clean in the sight of the general public when your relationship skills as a nurse are weak. Work on yourself and give out the best professional input and together we build and maintain a good reputation for the noble profession. Trust me; you will be the first person to enjoy it. Pass this information on by tapping the shoulders of a sister or brother of our own.

Do it for the sake of love.
I am one of your own,

*The Nurse-counselor.*

# CHAPTER *Five*

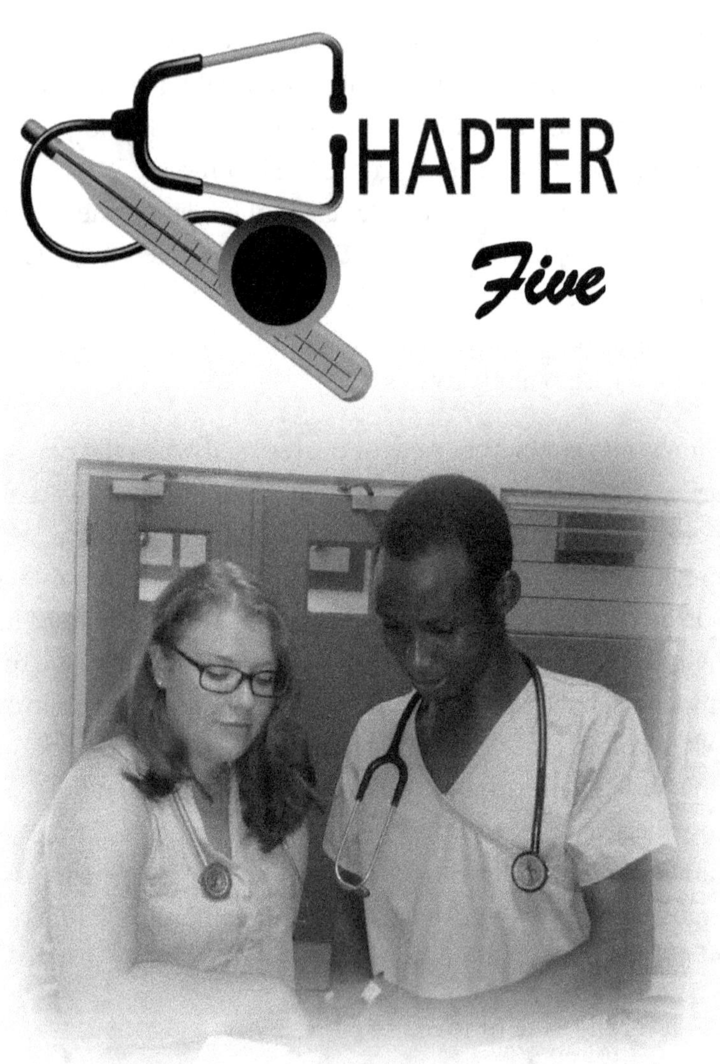

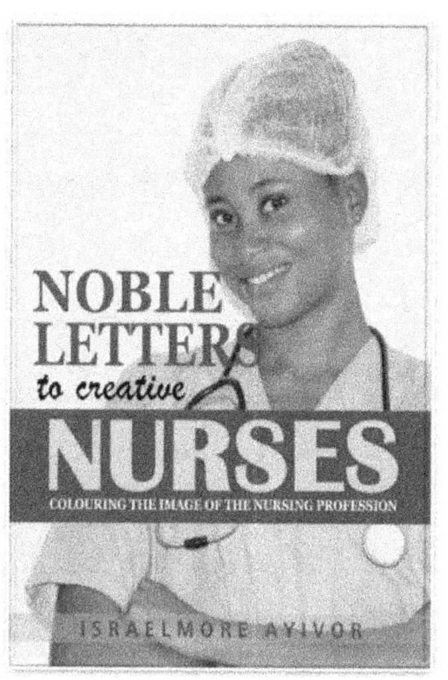

# NURSES AND THE LEGAL SYSTEM

*A letter from*
*The Law-Room*

<u>**To you, my unknown midwife!**</u>

*I don't know how I was born on earth*
*Only my midwife can tell how I made it here*
*I learnt it was a journey of life and death*
*I could not do it myself, I wasn't even aware*

*The first hands that gently handled my calm body*
*Did a very honourable job I grew up to know*
*When I was nobody, you were my somebody*
*My mother's severe pain, you made it low*

*I cried my first cry 'cause you gave me a surprise*
*I am thankful for the cares of your hands I felt*
*You don't receive it, but you deserve a prize*
*You deserve, I think a noble belt*

*I was too young to say "thank you" with honour*
*I urinated on you, but you didn't make it a case*
*Sorry for my delay through the stages of labour*
*Thank you for waiting on me till I showed my face*

*You were my coach on my way to victory*
*And you celebrated with me when I finally made it*
*You guided my steps until my birth became a history*
*I love you so much and still wonder how you did it*

---

Israelmore Ayivor

*Dear Nurse,*

I am here again with epistles of reminders. A quick one; I know you're aware the law guides your action as a nurse. You work within standards laid down. There is nothing like "this is the way I do it". If that "way" is not within the standard, you are inviting trouble to dine with you with contaminated hands. By-passing the standards and doing what the law frowns on is an effort to destroy the image and reputation of nursing. My lecturer always advices us that the nurse holds the keys to the courtrooms and when she decided that it shall not open, it will not open.

---

Have you ever wondered how the planet earth would be if there are no laws but there is an increase in crimes? Ungovernable! It would be totally ungovernable. You would never love to live in it; me neither. Fugitive files of atrocities would pile on one another until we begin to think about tidying up another planet for quick relocation. Everyone would take the "law" into their own hands and do anything, anyhow and to anyone and at anytime, anywhere. There is law, not to scare people to feel intimidated when they become aware of it, but rather to minimize crime and protect the vulnerable. Law guides everyone and nobody is above the constitution of the nation.

Members of the health team, including nurses are no exemptions when understanding and application of the law is mentioned. Nurses' actions are regulated by the law and a breach in the regulations may make your trends of actions to be considered as a crime. For this reason, I stand in the law room, though my brain has not been subjected to such a luminary training, to report to you what I have seen and heard and advice you the nurse that you should be careful of how you go about your work. Otherwise, you may think you are doing your best, yet you may still be liable if found going against the law. It doesn't matter whether you have knowledge of the law or not, if you breach it, you may be liable. Ignorance of the law is no excuse, they say. Treat this letter with care and thank me later.

Primarily what the nurse has to know about the law includes any information that answers the questions;

- Why was the law written?
- How was the law written?
- How is the law enforced?

I understand that the law wasn't created to harm anyone. It was rather created to protect us by giving us the opportunity to demonstrate acceptable behaviour. It is when you break the law that you will become an offender to face the full rigors of it. However, if you don't break the law, the law remains your friend and personal advisor. The law achieves five (5) main principles;

**Harm principle:** The law protects us from harm. Anyone who tries to harm us becomes liable.

**Parent principle:** The law acts as our parent, guiding our actions and characters.

**Morality principle:** The law regulates the norms of society by telling what's right and what's wrong.

**Donation principle:** The law also advocates for the needy and the less privilege in the society.

**Static principle:** The law creates a standard or status quo for society. It serves as a yardstick for measuring varying degrees of good things and bad things.

Now the main purpose why I am writing this particular letter is to re-inform nurses to be alert and keep their knowledge and practice at professional levels in order to avoid trampling their hardworking pairs of feet into the gloomy consequences of lawful sentences. A nurse may be sued when suspected to be liable. Suing the nurse does not necessarily mean she has committed the crime. When the case is tried, that is when the grandiose superiority of the law and the supreme art of the justice system will reveal it.

There is no need for the nurse to panic when sued if she believes what she has done is right. It means as long as you have been doing what is right, being sued should not make you sick and scared. What I just want to say is that when a nurse is accused, it doesn't mean she is necessarily wrong unless it has been proven. Sometimes the duty may exist, nurse may take a certain action, but when the action taken and the harm caused are not related, the nurse will be vindicated. However relating the law to the nursing profession, sometimes a mere accusation is taken as breakage of the law and may drag the reputation of the profession into muddy waters warmed with impotent humiliations.

The perceptions  of general public sometimes makes me wonder if they have an issue with nursing and they're just waiting for something tiny to come out as an a legal issue so they can put their magnifying glasses on it. News about legal issues pertaining to nursing seems to travel far and long. People would say all manner of things as if nurses are enemies even if the issue goes through the legal system and found the nurse faultless. When the rumour breaks out about the bad act of the nurse, it travels faster. When it is later found to be untrue, nobody circulates that one. This is the reason why it would be very good for the nurse not to be interested in fighting to win cases leveled against them, but to do all they can to avoid creating an opportunity for a case to be made against them.

I walked out of my nurse manager's office recently with so much inspiration. She informed me briefly after I submitted my report for cross-examination and marking. In her words, she acknowledge that if a nurse should do thousand things which are right and one thing which is not right, that one thing can be used to discredit the thousand things she did very well. She added that the only way some people can admire and appreciate the work of nurses is when they are made to watch the video coverage of nurses attending to patient with passion when they are not around. For the sake of privacy, you don't see the work nurses do behind the scenes. It is done behind the scenes and it is perceived as if nothing has been done.

Nursing is not like football where the match is shown live and general public knows how strong the opponents are, who scores, who dribbles very well or who isn't well trained. Nursing is not like journalism where everyone can tell whether the story being reported is coherent and congruent. When the newscaster is fluent, everyone behind the TV can testify about it. Nursing is not like that. The real practices happen behind closed-doors and are unseen. And so you don't have to be surprise when the hard "unseen" work is not appreciated. The writer reporting from the law room urges nurses to know the law guiding their work. The nurses must invest into knowing the legal implications of the roles they play as civil servants. Ignorance of the law is self-imprisonment in advance.

That reminds me of my school days. I met a man who came back to the facility I was being trained in few days after discharge. He came for checkup. His review day was not due, but he came to do some tests voluntarily. It all happened when one of the nurses who managed him while he was on admission was accused of malpractice on another patient. The news broke strong fences and travelled wide and when he heard it, he wanted to check if everything was alright with him since that nurse also worked on him before. That was why he returned to request that the doctor orders some laboratory tests to be sure if he was also not treated wrongfully.

The stigma attached to being found guilty alone is difficult to be handled especially by people who have emotional issues. Once you have gone through and have that label on you, even your own colleagues will not trust you if their families or friends are in your care. Everyone would want to be sure you are not doing that mistake again. One time you are welcomed and another time, you are doubted; you may end up living your career life between fluctuations of commendations and condemnations. You won't love it. However, if you are known to be competent by yourself and others, happiness will forever sing itself in memory of you.

To avoid having legal issues;

Always inform the patient concerning procedures you want to do and convey to him the essence of doing that procedure. If the patient cannot respond, inform his relatives and gain their consent.

Explain the possible side effects of the drugs you have been instructed to give. If you don't explain the side effects and they occur, the patient may misinterpret it as a sign of your negligence. Negligence could be in "not giving a care" and "not giving information".

Never share personal information of patients to another patient or your friends or the people your patient would never want to have access to such information.

Ensure the patient signs the consent form for any invasive procedure to be performed. Also, gain the patient's consent before you carry out a procedure that would have his private body part exposed partially or fully.

Don't force a patient in his right senses to take a medicine he refused to take if the patient is an adult. The patient has the right to refuse your care and when that happens, you just have to document your facts and be safe.

Before you agree to let the patient's wrong choices rule, explain to him the consequences of his choices. For instance if a patient refuses to take his medicine, don't just stand on that and decide not to give it. Explain deeper. When he insists, accept his choice and make a record of it.

Document all your nursing procedures in the nurse's notes for referencing when necessary. Your nurses' notes should be simple but should not be too abbreviated to be devoid of facts that can defend you sooner or later. Your handwriting should be readable by another person. I trust you know all these tips. I'm just giving you catalogue of reminders.

Keep the nurses note safely. If you have to staple or clip, do it neatly and avoid supplementary sheets from falling off. For the sake of legal issues, I think suggestions concerning "nurses' folder" should be taken seriously so we can do away with using insecure leaflets or supplementary sheets very soon. A "folder for nurses", my lecturer in one of her passionate lectures said would be of a great help than pieces of papers that makes the documents clumsy. I agree and I know if you agree, someone else also agrees, we should advocate for "nurses' folder". It would help the nurse, the Health facility and the Health Service.

Be honest. Never write anything you did not do and do anything you would not write. Don't write things you did not do in order to be seen as a hard working staff. Sometimes the evidences of the work you did and the work you do not do are going to stare in your face and you may not be able to defend it there. For instance, take it that a certain nurse didn't do suturing of a wound on a certain patient's forehead, but she documented it. In years to come, one can tell whether suturing was done at the forehead of a person or not. The stitches' marks will prove it and if there is nothing to show what you have written, you may not be trusted in another case involving your so-called sincere documentation.

Upgrade your knowledge often so that you don't use archaic knowledge and skills to manage any patient. When a patient discovers that you are not using up-to-date information to care for him, he may take you on. For instance, administering drugs that have been withdrawn and replaced after they have been found to be less effective is a critical example. It is not enough the Doctor knows it. You too must know the current medical management of the diagnosis you are managing.

Two things you can't forget;

**Read the patients' charter and be informed concerning the details it captures.**

**Read the code of ethics of nursing written by your employer and ensure you understand them.**

Nurses can fall victims of many legal concessions called Tort Laws. A tort, in common law jurisdictions, is a civil wrong that unfairly causes someone else to suffer loss or harm resulting in legal liability for the person who commits the tortious act. The person who commits the tortious act is called a tortfeasor. (Wikipedia, 2017). A tort could be intentional or unintentional. Some examples of torts include but not limited to; defamation, assault, battery, larceny, invasion of privacy, malpractice and negligence.

Still on my desire to remind you, I would like to take you through the two most common tort laws a nurse is usually liable to and provide possible examples where breaches are made for your own use.

**Negligence:**

A person can be said to be guilty of Tort of Negligence when there is a duty she must fulfill but did not fulfill it. For example;

- Starving a patient who needs to be fed with food.
- Not being able to inform a patient of procedures he needs to be aware of and give his consent to.
- Not giving a medication a patient is due to receive.

**Malpractice:**

A person is said to be guilty of Tort of Malpractice when a person performs a duty wrongly or performs a wrong duty. For example;

- Giving medications at the wrong time, or giving wrong medications, or wrong doses of right medications.
- Performing procedures which are not part of your job description (e.g. a nurse carrying out Caesarian Section).

- Not monitoring vital signs of patients to notice a change in condition.

Now when you study a little portion of the law, you will discover that before the claim of a patient is justified, it goes through a legal process. Legal elements would be used to check if the claim is true. Most times the nurse is vindicated and that has to do with the outcome of the test of the claim with the legal elements. I learnt that four legal elements are used;

1. **Duty:** Has the duty of care existed?
2. **Breach:** Has the nurse breached the duty?
3. **Damages:** Are there damages caused?
4. **Causative:** Is the damage linked to the breach?

When a nurse did not explain to patient the possible side effects of a certain drug and the patient eventually experiences some uncomfortable changes in his body, the patient can raise negligence claim. However, that claim can hold water if it passes the test with the legal elements. So in an instance where the nurse is vindicated, a possible outcome could be;

1. **Duty:** The nurse gave the medicine (eye drop).
2. **Breach:** She did not educate the patient on the side effects of the medicine.
3. **Damages:** The patient started having abdominal pains.
4. **Causative:** The harm (abdominal pain) is not linked to the duty breached (not educating the patient on side effects of the eye drop before giving it).

Legal issues are serious and the nurse should not take them for granted. The earlier we know and avoid even a mere accusation, the better. That is why the writer of this letter is of the view that every nurse should become a self-acclaimed lawyer, knowing the law guiding her practice off-head. I am aware there may be people who are always opening their eyes wide to find faults and make legal issues out of the work of hard working nurses. As a nurse, just make sure that you do the right thing and you will be safe no matter how many times your work has been reviewed.

Legal issue could easily lead to great damages to a person's reputation, financial loss to the facility or the individual involved and above all, possible closure of the facility and in critical cases, a seizure of licenses used for practicing by the nurse involved. Let's do our best to be on course.

In conclusion, dear nurse, I charge you to read more on legal matters involving health care locally, nationally and internationally. Learn from the consequences and the results of those who have been found liable and advice yourself. However, do not be so afraid of the law in such a way that you forget the joy hidden in caring for people. You are not just giving nursing cares in order to obey laws, but rather to achieve the aim of alleviating pain and promoting health. Do it right, not just because the law requires it, but also because there is joy in rendering good services. Together, we shall send a pure colour of the image of nursing to the world by doing what is required.

*From the law-room,* With Kind regards.

# CHAPTER
## Six

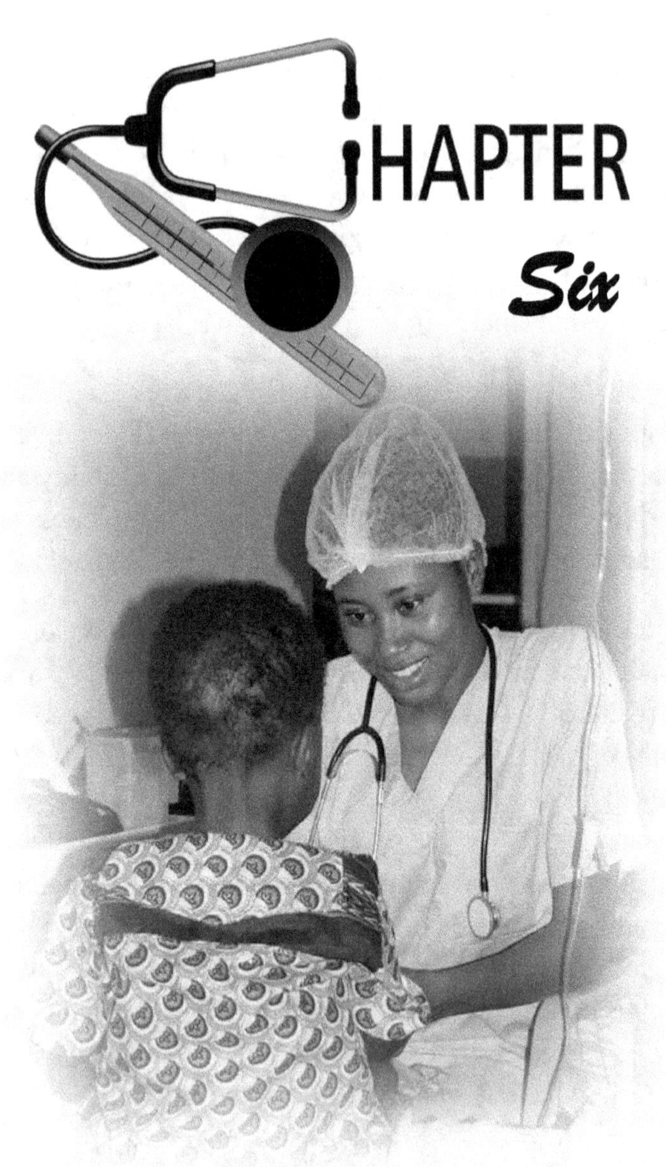

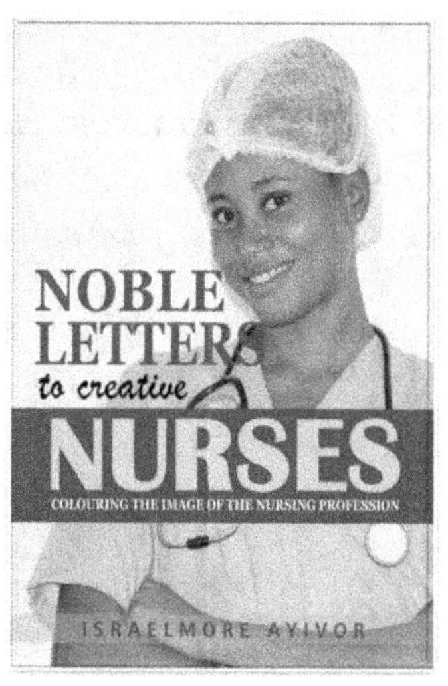

# YOUR LIFETSYLE IS A NURSING TOOL

*A letter from*
*The Lifestyle Teacher*

# <u>The lifestyle of the nurse</u>

*Your words may convince so many people*
*But your actions make them to trust you*
*It is a simple lesson to keep; very simple*
*Give your best in everything you do*

*Make sure your life is a great source of credit*
*Always to Nursing, your profession*
*If it is not so now, it's not too late, you can edit*
*Get up now and start making a resolution*

*You are the eyes of sight for the blind*
*You are the ears of hearing for the deaf*
*Your lifestyle must tell you are very kind*
*Be careful about how you live your life*

*Don't discriminate because of tribe or race*
*Not even religion, politics or colour of the face*
*Love every human being, whites and blacks*
*No matter whether he is rich or he lacks*

*You may not be honoured with a big award*
*Look not there; that isn't your reward*
*The clean image of the nursing profession*
*Is the number one reward for your devotion*

Israelmore Ayivor

*Dear Nurse*, Your lifestyle is like a paint brush on the wall of the nursing profession. If your lifestyle is bad, the profession is seen as bad by people who know your name attached to the nursing profession. When your life is attractive, the profession becomes attractive. Think about this. The fact that you made a choice to become a nurse means you can't live life anyhow. Whatever you do or say whether in uniform or not in uniform can mend or destroy the image of nursing.

---

I am writing these letters to you from the comfort of my table. However, I am of the view that this particular type is very important among them all. I treasured the ink used to scribe this letter because I have no doubt that it is the ink destined to right many wrongs. Please, treat this letter with diligence because the pictorial view of your lifestyle after work and outside the hospital seems to have a familiar affiliation with the contents it harbours. I entitle it; "your lifestyle is a nursing tool". If you find that title to be too casual, you can make your own titles out of it; "Your behaviour is a healing factor" or "How you act, determines how your patient responds to the sickness he brought" or "How you live, is how nursing lives."

Your lifestyle is collectively determined by many factors in or outside your knowledge. However, two main factors seem to be playing dominant roles to tell who you truly are and why you are such a person, behaving in such a way. They are; your attitude and your actions. Your attitude creates the path and your actions drag you on it. When your attitude is crooked, your actions may not enjoy a journey on the path it creates. Also, when your actions are wayward, they will not make use of the path your attitude creates.

**Your attitude:**

Attitude is simply defined as a way of thinking about something or the perception someone carries about something which influence his/her actions. It is a feeling or opinion of someone that influences his/her behaviour. For instance, someone may think "anyone who corrects me hates me." When this becomes an attitude, it influences the person's behaviour. In that sense, he/she may not want to get closer to anyone who tries to offer him/her corrections based on certain issues.

Two people can experience the same situation and develop two different attitudes from it. For instance, a regulation, say "come to work early" can generate two different perceptions and hence cultivate two different lifestyles. While one nurse thinks "when I come to work early, I have more work to do and I will be very tired, so let me delay", another nurse may think, "When I come to work early, I will do much work early and become a bit free towards the end of my shift, so let me go early." You can predict that a lazy nurse would be born out of the former attitude and a diligent nurse, out of the later. Attitude for that matter helps us to make choices; right or wrong.

**Your actions:**

Actions are born out of attitudes. A negative attitude is likely to breed a negative action and vice versa. However, we can't be sure that a bad attitude will always make the nurse to behave in awkward matter due to other factors that might come to play. A good attitude alone is a good environment for a good behaviour, but other factors can alter the consequent action to become otherwise. I will tell you why.

A nurse whose attitude makes her lazy may end up working hard when Nurse Manager (or a supervisor) is on her supervision duty. At this point, she works because she doesn't want to be queried. This is another bad attitude though, but at least, it hasn't affected the work she does. And if you care to know the attitude, it is that thinking that "work has to be done to avoid punishment", instead of "work has to be done to alleviate pain and promote health." With the wrong attitude, the work is done because the person responsible for the punishment is present in the ward. The presence of the Nurse Manager in the ward, hence does not serve as a motivation, but as a threat to the lazy nurse. Nurse Managers are not left out. The negative attitude I am writing on at times, is also displayed by some Nurse Managers during the course of their supervision duties. Though is it helpful to find faults, I think fault-finding should not be the sole plan and purpose for supervision. Finding faults at times may leave the nurses to work under threats. I may be wrong, but I think sometimes, finding ways to motivation someone for a good thing done is enough to encourage the person to correct other wrong things usually done.

Back to the point; "Lifestyle vs. nursing goals". You want to remember the title of this letter again; "your lifestyle is a nursing tool". I remember vividly the story of a woman who told me she decided never to step into the premises of the hospital in her hometown for review against her hypertensive condition. She defaulted the treatment and started developing complications at home. Her story among many other stories was the condition that even pushed me to pick up my pen to write to you. Simply, she refused to visit the hospital because of how she was treated by a certain nurse. Perhaps thinking she may be treated the same way, she insisted that as long as that nurse is still working in the hospital, she won't come around. She just doesn't want to see her.

Don't hurriedly blame her for her way of thinking. Maybe you want to say she isn't serious. Or you want to conclude that if she loves herself, she would visit the hospital against all odds. It is obvious she also has a crooked attitude and that attitude made her to pick that choice. However, this letter is not written to correct the patient's attitude. It is a letter to nurses and not patients. Sorry, the Lifestyle Teacher has to descend on only the nurse, and not the patient. Do you know that in the above scenario, the lifestyle of the nurse was responsible for the patient's refusal to come to the hospital? Do you know, moments after discharge, impressions created by a nurse follows the patients home and can determine if they would seek to use the same facility again? One encounter with a patient can continue making impacts in his life even after the resolution phase of Hildegard Paplau's interpersonal relationship theory.

Let me quickly refer you to some of the lovely lines of the solemn Nurses' Pledge;

**"I acknowledge that the special training I have received has prepared me as a responsible member of the community…"**

A responsible member of the community will never get involved in committing vices. A responsible member of the society will not treat a patient in the ward in such a way that when he goes back to the same community after work, she would not be accepted or welcomed.

**"I promise that my personal life shall at all times bring credit to my profession…"**

Your personal life is essential because even out of work, people will refer to you as "nurse". You are known as a nurse in the ward and when you close from work, you are not known as a police, but still as a nurse. It means when you do something good, people will say, "that's the nurse", "that's the midwife." Same way when you do something bad, people will point fingers saying, "did you see that nurse?" Even if the manner in which you behaved and what you did is not related to health care, your "nursing" background is attached and attacked when people know you to be one.

When a patient knows a certain nurse to be an addicted smoker, it would take a divine intervention to inform the patient to accept knowledge on prevention of liver cirrhosis when receiving education on it. The truth is that your personal life will tell if people should trust your instructions or not. You can change the life of people indirectly by how you behave. They just see your good works and give the reverence to the nursing profession whose image is almost sunken.

A study conducted on nursing image as a profession indicated that the public image of nursing and the media portrayal of nursing are the greatest factors that have negative influence on the nursing image (Fauda, Sleem & Mohammed, 2016). In order to redeem the falling image, the nurses must work hard to avoid the media from getting evidences to argue out their so-called suspicions. The genuine way for preventing those evidences is by acting right. However, when the lifestyle of the nurse keeps repelling people away, these are the people who would feed the media to paint the dirty image about the profession.

I am of the view that nurses are respected based on their character and not on their knowledge. I am not discrediting the essence of nurses to be knowledgeable, but I am sure most patients do not know much about the care they need. So when the nurse is not knowledgeable, they don't even know it. However, when the nurse is rude, careless, rowdy, proud, arrogant, and impatient and lacks self-control, the patient will know it. The same way when the nurse is lovely, cheerful, understanding, caring, polite, compassionate, empathetic, patient, humble, dependable and courteous, the patient will know. The attitude and actions of the nurse is what reveals these traits and when these traits are revealed; it goes ways to give not only the nurse involved, but also "nursing" in general a specific negative brand.

I understand that there are times when the nurse must ensure discipline in the ward and never compromise to see things go wrong. For instance, you don't see family members of patients crowded in the ward and allow them to make noise, and disturb the patient's sleep pattern. To them, they are doing the patients a favour by visiting him, but to your nursing care plan, they may be doing the wrong thing by disrupting the patient's sleep pattern.

It means you have to explain to them politely on how the essence of they keeping away from the patient for the mean time. You could encourage them humbly that they can return during visiting hours. I believe the way and manner in which you say this to them will either make them respond to you in peace or create tension by exchanging words with you. Sometimes, family members may request for discharge of patient since they can no longer trust some nurses because of their choices of words. When a customer feels humiliated, insulted, and belittled, he may not wish to do business with you. However, when the person feels appreciated, encouraged and satisfied, he would wish to maintain an established relationship for future services. Take note of this and when you are building a therapeutic relationship, let your lifestyle create a deeper trust.

Take note of this fact that everything you do in your society contributes to adding or subtracting credit from the nursing profession. Wherever you are, be careful what you do or say. Be careful of how you talk or react. Be careful of what you advice people on and what you are seen doing yourself. All these and many more factors make you a good nurse even when you are not wearing the nursing uniform. The beautiful image of nursing is not hiding in the equipments, bed accessories and the serenity of the health facility. It is in the quality of life the nurse lives. Live a positive life that would make people willing to receive care from you anytime they need you. And never forget this; you are not doing the patient any favour. The patient is rather doing you a favour by giving you the chance for you to work on him. Stay blessed and let your light shine to the general public, that they may see your selfless efforts and give respect to nursing which is your profession.

Do more; achieve more. Thank you for giving me your attention.

*The Lifestyle Teacher.*

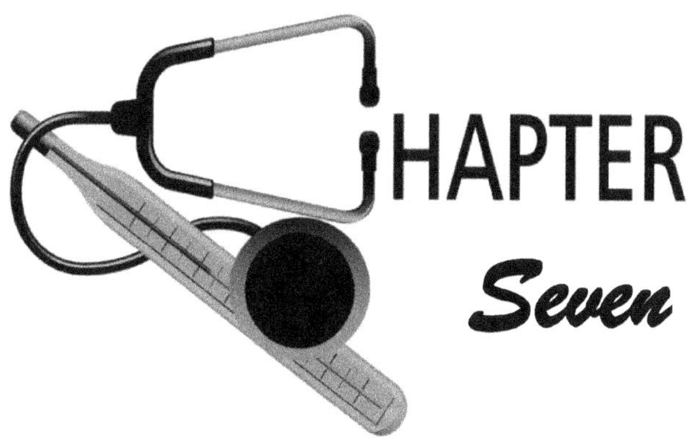

CHAPTER
Seven


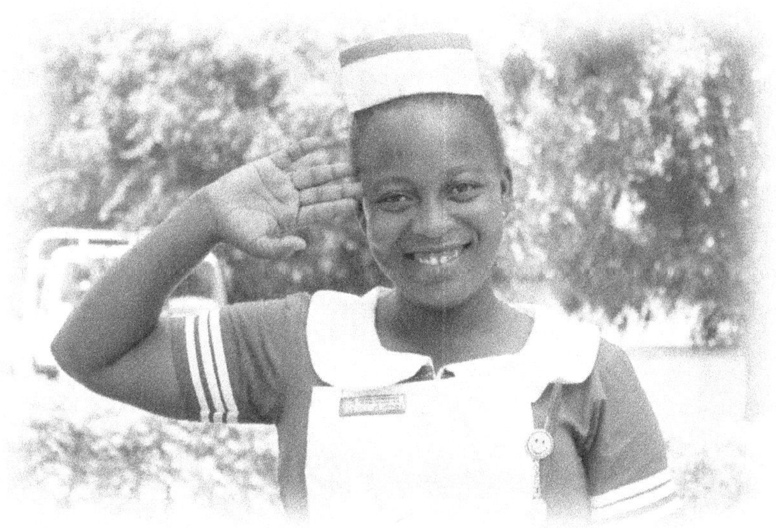

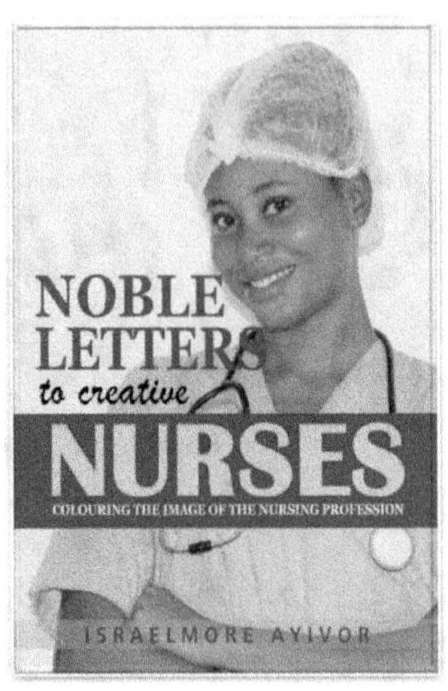

# AN OPEN LETTER TO NURSING STUDENTS

*A letter from the
student nurse alumnus*

Beside a beautiful graveyard, an inscription was mounted. It reads, "We were once like you. You will also be like us." The inmates of the cemetery seem to be responsible for this piece of information. They claim they were once alive, kicking, walking, talking and smiling like us. And definitely, we the living, when we die, will also find our homes under the sandy layers of the earth. The student nurse will one day become a staff when her schooling years die off. She would be ushered into a new edifice of career life with no hard training, less instructions, no academic examinations, no group presentation, no clinical assessments, etc. Some are of the view that once their academic years are over and they begin to work, they would earn freedom. But is that true? Is there a relief in physical exertion and stress when you stop becoming a student? Is there more comfort in being a staff than being a student? Time will tell!

---

With all due respect, this letter is addressed to all nursing students, known and unknown, old or young, native or foreigner, male or female, pursing certificate, diploma, degree programmes. You are the protégés in the profession and without you, there shall be no more nursing in a short time to come. You are like the bud, yet to become flowers and then we talk about fruits. I have no time on my side, so I want to start my lengthy letter quickly with the twin questions. They are questions I struggled to find answers to. Maybe you can be of help, I guess. So I ask;

**Question 1:** Does time and experience change the attitude of a person?

**Question 2:** Does experience influence the behaviour and character of a person?

If it doesn't, then why was I surprised? And if it does, how does it do it? I ask these questions because I was dumbfounded. I was dumbfounded with a harmless but horrible experience. An experience that left me thinking if "time" can be responsible for change of lifestyle and behaviour. I met a surprise in my life and in the face of this surprise; I am close to getting confused and I need a help. Let me share this story with you and after it, I will come back to my questions again. I treasure these questions because I believe they carry stars; Stars to drive away the darkness lingering around the annals of our noble profession. Please, read my story with patience.

We were school mates. We studied and worked as students in the same ward before. I got to know her. She knew me too. I came into her life at the very time she needed me. Yes. I knew what she needed and that was what I gave. She was so happy, I became so happy, everyone around was happy, except the devil because his plans did not work out.

If you care to know, it was late in the evening when she left the ward without asking permission from our superiors and went to buy food outside the yard to deal with her hunger. It was forbidden for a nursing student to leave the ward

without receiving an authorization from a superior while on
duty. She broke the rule. She deserved the punishment. At
least, a caution would do; perhaps for this incidence being
her first offence. The senior nurse, our supervisor got to
notice that she broke the rule. She became very furious and
could not tolerate that lawless style of life. With red hot
eyes, she was waiting patiently for the potential culprit to
return; ready to give out what I think had been the thickest
punishment to be handled by a disobedient student nurse in
that week. We all knew this senior. She never saw nonsense
and overlooked it. If you want to sweat under air condition,
just try to be stubborn; she would drill that hole into you
and pick out that tissue of indiscipline which makes you
behave the way you do.

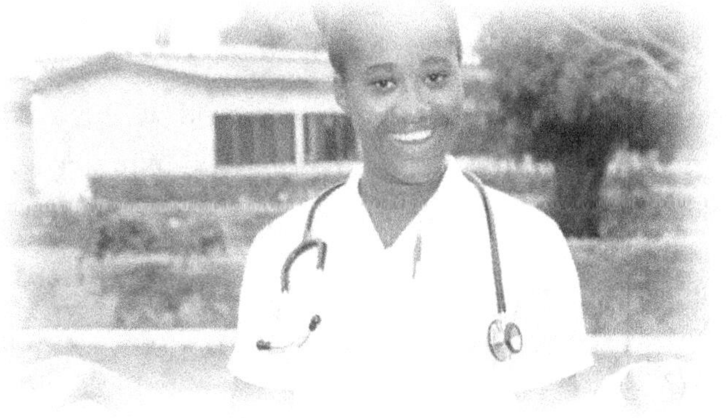

Alas! The door opened. Here comes the much awaited
culprit. "Come here!", she retorted. "Disobedient girl!",
said added. "Stop there!"; she came again. "Don't you have
ears?". She roared. The student nurse became terrified, sad
and appeared miserably frustrated. She doesn't know

whether to move forward or remain static because "come here" and "stop there" came as identical twin sisters from the lion-voice of the furious nurse. But she thought faster about "don't you have ears?" and that statement pushed her to get closer.

In front of patients, their relatives and other nurses and junior nurses, I inclusive, this student nurse was drilled, screwed and disgraced for her offence and her next off-day was cancelled because she left the ward +without permission. With both hands at her back (as a sign of respect) and head bend as if she was admiring the glossy nature of the cemented floor (as a result of humiliation); she saturated her cheeks with tears. I consoled her hours after and encourage her to wipe her tears. I was beside her to prevent her from thinking negatively. I spoke nice words to her and pampered her to make her feel welcomed. I was preventing her from emotional breakdown. I gave her a surprise escort to her house after work and we engaged in conversations that made her forgot the sad experience. My trick worked. She became happy again!

If you care to know, we all completed the training school and were distributed to various hospitals. We never met again years and months after. Then one day, I was sick in the town where she worked. I came for a religious conference to honour an invitation as a motivational speaker and there, the ailment took my abdomen by surprise. I assisted myself to the hospital nearest hospital in the town. I went to one of the wards to introduce myself to any nurse that maybe on duty. Unfortunately, when I opened the gate of the ward, the door slipped off my hands and slammed with a loud noise. Immediately, I heard a shout from a distance; "what's the problem?"; "who is there?", "are you a villager?", "are you not civilized?"; "don't you know how to open doors gently?". The voice added several severely annoying words, but the final one I can remember was very long. The voice said that; "don't bring your home behaviours here. When you go to Rome, do what Romans do. Only ignorant and uncivilized people slam doors that way."

I was sad but I went closer and closer. The image of the person pouring those bullets was getting focused by my eye lenses. Sharp! I was able to identify the nurse who spewed those words at me. She didn't change so much! If you care to know, she was that very person who was humiliated with corrosive words by the older nurse when we were students. Oh okay, you now grow wings and horns, I imagined. She recognized me, and I could read regrets forming dark clouds on her eyes. Was she regretting those words she spoke to me when she wasn't aware I was the person who entered? Yes! She was very shy and wanted to apologize, but her lips refused to help her out. Her lips rioted epileptically and never gave her chances to talk.

Well, back to the question I kept thinking about; "does time and experience change attitude and character?" Which one does that job? Time or experience or both? I ask this question because I saw a change of lifestyle. Someone who was treated with abusive words by a staff when she was in school and she felt the pain, when she became a staff, also treats other people with abusive words.

- What could be the cause?
- When did the change happen?
- How did she become the very person she hated to work with?
- How did she turn to become the very person who made her cried?

My further investigation revealed that she was the staff feared by student nurses and midwives most since she drills holes in them to pick out tissues of indiscipline, doing so in ways uncomfortable to the to-be-nurses and to-be-midwives. Perhaps she made some student nurses also cried. And what is the fate of those students who also dislike her way of life? Would they also become like her when time unfolds and experience wins their hearts?

When Promise Ogochukwu, a Nigerian author, held the hand of that fresh baby born in the maternity ward, she was in doubt about her future. If you read the first chapter of her book "Wild letters in harmattan", you will understand what I mean. It is a must read, I believe. When you see a new born baby, she always looks innocent, harmless and cheerful with puffy cheeps, softer lips, spotless skin and fresh gums. When you take your eyes off and remember the pastors, lawyers, teachers, nurses, politicians, thieves, rapists, racists, footballers, musicians, pornographers, etc., you shouldn't be wrong to think they were all once like the innocent, fresh and harmless baby.

And looking at the harmless baby, nobody can tell who among the above list she would become. However, definitely, who she becomes is a sign that something happened along the line as she grows up. All sorts of human beings; the proud, humble, principled, hardworking, polite, arrogant, heartless, wicked, friendly, bold, greedy, tactless, cunning, rough, ignorance, frightful, teachable, corruptible, covetous, jealous, generous, peaceful, and more; they were born innocent and harmless and when they were babies, no one could tell who they would become. (Ogochukwu, 2009).

During our orientation week in the nursing school, I remember we were taken to the mortuary on a particular day to see how corpses are preserved. Some students wept after going through the mortuary cold room. Others lost their appetite for food and water because of the reality of the experience. I am not sure those who cried by then would cry today when they go through the same experience. Why won't they cry again? Because of experience? Because of familiarity? Because of an inactivated conscience? Because death is now normal? The answer may vary from person to person.

You may not be able to tell the fate of student nurses until they begin to work as staff nurses. Sometimes, those who were lazy student nurses become hard working staff nurses. Other times those who were active initially begin to lose their passion and become lazy after graduation. Something definitely must have happen on the way. It is difficult to tell how. It is not easy to know when. However, I charge all student nurses to be vibrant and never attempt to quench the light of passion they harbour; but rather they should add more fuel so it can keep burning.

My personal observation indicate that most student nurses absent themselves from work without permission while others habitually report to work late. Others are eager to close and go home while some also exhibit all forms of laziness when it is time for them to assist in carrying out tasks. Though there is still a wholesome number that shows commitment and are prepared to learn with humility and politeness, still there is a big fraction that stands on familiarity with staffs to misbehave. The image of Nursing as a profession is close to the grave when students being raised do not prove to the world they are capable of taking the batons and running the race better.

My personal experience revealed to me that when some student nurses become close friends to some staffs, they begin to use that opportunity to fool and misbehave. When this happens it becomes difficult for the staff to give out the necessary punishment to the student when she offends. On the other hand, students who are given deserving punishments by staffs they have become familiar with tend to openly refuse to do the punishment. They think they are co-equals with the workers they become familiar with. A research conducted by Dorothy Awua-Peasah, Linda Akuamoah Sarfo and Florence Asamoah in 2013 on "the attitudes of student nurses toward clinical work" indicates that, Nursing students who are absent during clinical working hours or report late to clinical work are likely to miss out on important learning opportunities." with reference to the their targets, they also concluded that;

"Even though, the nursing students attended general rounds, they did not embark on the opportunity to interact and learn from the medical staff by asking questions. Some of the students were nervous during clinicals, but anxiety in the clinicals negatively impedes students' learning." (Dorothy Awua-Peasah, Linda Akuamoah Sarfo, 2013). I talked to some nursing students and I am convinced that the nervousness most students exhibit is as a result of the fear of being ridiculed when they ask unwise questions on ward rounds or answer right questions the wrong way. Some are also frightened because of the attitude of the staff they are on duty with.

The impatient attitude of some staffs also end up making lots of students to regret their choices of taking the nursing course. When I used to be a student nurse on Clinicals in a certain hospital, I always wanted to watch the time table to know when I would be on duty with a certain nurse. On the days I had to run duties with this nurse, I spent the more hours in the bathroom than usual; not because I wanted to have a fair skin, but because while I bathed to go work, I kept thinking about how horrible the day would be for me. I went through though and I am writing this letter to you, in+ order to encourage you to persevere and go through.

The three researchers also observed that, the attitude of first year students' towards care is always better than that of their final year counterparts, citing the reason to be the tension imposed on them by the challenges of sitting for the licensing examinations. This makes them not to take clinical work very serious. (Awua-Peasah, et. al. 2013). Another thing I think is responsible for the lackadaisical attitude of student nurses in their final years is familiarity with the work. Some think they already know most procedures, so they see no reason to be present and active during clinical sessions. Finally, I think another serious area to look at should be the way most nursing students use mobile phone devices in the ward. Instead of using the phones to do researches on disease conditions they meet so they can read wide, most of them go wayward, misusing this opportunity. Aside fidgeting with the phones on social media pleasures while serious cares need to be rendered, some even go taking pictures while carrying out procedure without gaining the consents of the patients. Most of the students who do that are yet to grasp knowledge on the legal implications of their acts.

As a student nurse,

- Be determined that you will be the correction of what you have seen going wrong. If you don't like something, correct it and don't copy it. In the words of Mahatma Gandhi: "Be the change you wish to see." Just dare to be the change.

- Also remember, you may be treated the same way you treat your seniors when you also become a senior. Treat your seniors with respect if you want to be treated with respect and I know you want it.

- Report to work and ensure that you are always punctual. Habit formation is an easy thing, but breaking it becomes very difficult. Some of the bad habits that become difficult to change include lateness, complaining, over dependency on other staffs for the success of work and truancy.

Watch yourself when;

1. You hear every staff complaining about a particular thing you have been doing in a bad way.
2. Nobody wants to be on duty with you because of some obvious reason they have truly justified.
3. Your patient gives a directive that you should not be assigned to handle him again.
4. You discover that the spirit of passion for the work is leaving you slowly and slowly and it's being replaced by remorse.
5. You complain more than you encourage yourself. Complaints neither heal you nor your patient.
6. You begin to think you are better than other nursing students or staffs because you had better results in your End of Semester theory exams.

To conclude, I am so concerned about those of you who are overexcited and want changes to be made about what is done. I am aware some of you aren't happy with certain things as far practical Nursing is concerned and you vowed that when you step in the shoes of your forbearers, you would make changes. I plead with you, inasmuch as you are interested in change, you don't rather grow up and become worse. I admire your hot passion to work hard to redeem the falling image of Nursing as a career. However, be patient, thoughtful and wise. Your spirit and passion for changes should not die the moment you start taking salaries. The incoming of salary should not tune your mind to fall in love with the status quo.

To add to it, some of the things you think should be change, you will grow up soon to realize they are relevant and changing them would cause more havoc. You know, when you are fresh in the system, you are likely to argue everything out; "why are our tutors loading us with tutorials?", "our clinical in-charges have not given us much off days on the time table", "they are stressing us", "our exams are too hard", etc. You may even go to the extent of saying so many things concerning the Nursing and Midwifery regulatory bodies, and that excitement sometimes comes because you're not in that position to see what goes on.

I write from the ventricles of my heart to tell you that complaining too much won't make you a good nurse. What you are going through now perhaps is just tiny compared to what you will go through when you begin to practice. Save the time spent on those complaints and adjust yourself to cope. Nursing students are not the only people who undergo stress in their education. Have you thought of what petrochemical engineering students go through? Do you know how stressful Archeology can be? What about statistics? Maybe you should try them for just a week and see how they also taste. Perhaps you would beg to come back to the nursing you complained about.

Finally, please heed to my cry. I see something dangerous that happens in some Nursing School where different programmes are offered. Most times students offering

Diploma programmes think they're the best on campus while the others offering Certificate programmes are below their levels. Students offering Certificate programmes think they're being looked down upon and while some of the begin to feel inferior within themselves; others dare to raise shoulders to contest over equality. This sometimes ends in arguments and controversies further leading to fights and lots of beefs here and there. That's abominable and I think students who engage in these beefs aren't intelligent! Please, these kinds of News are not good for my health. Anytime I hear of them, I experience running stomach… I am even having nausea right now. I will stop my letter here.

To end this letter, I want to charge you once more. If you are excited to make a change, let not the fire of your excitement change when you get to the very place you need to be to make such a change. However, don't dream of making a change on something that is already working. Do enjoy your studies and see you one day becoming an agent of positive change.

Best regards,
*A former student nurse.*

# CHAPTER
## *Seven*

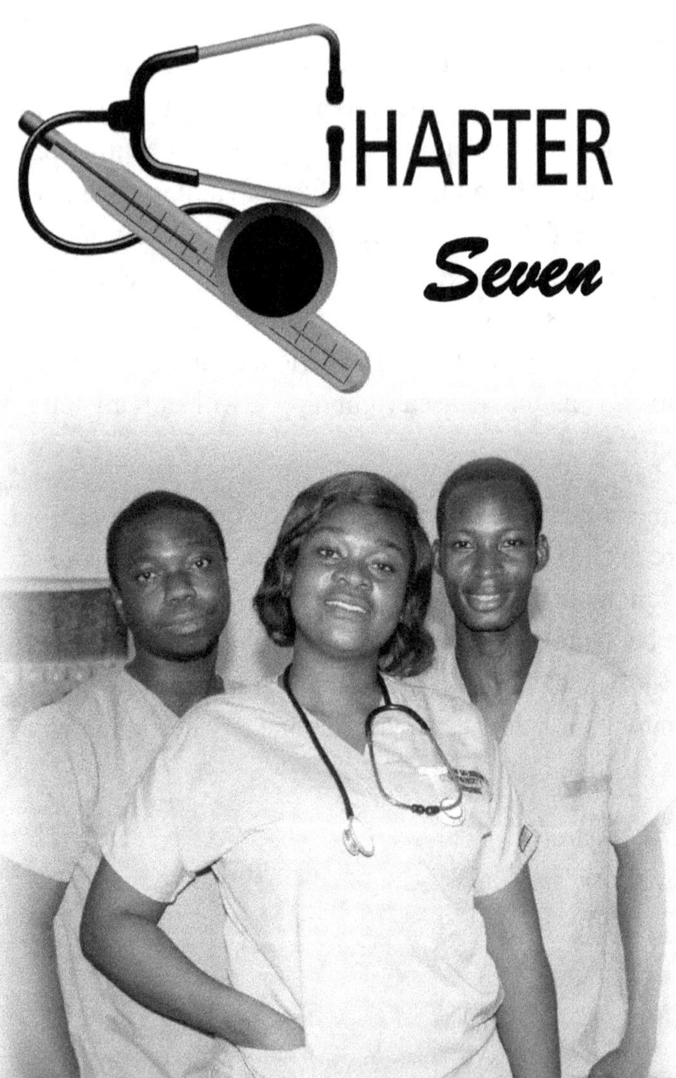

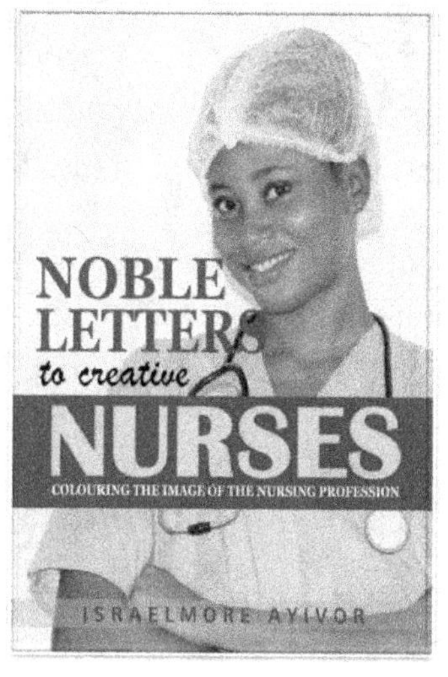

# QUOTES
# FOR NURSES

*Dear nurse,*

I am so mindful that the work you do is not easy. Most of your hard works are done in secret and you have no gut to boast about it. The other day, I watched a trained teacher on T.V who openly talked about one of his students who became great a great entrepreneur. These were his words;

"He was my taught. I taught him in primary school. I taught him mathematics. He was an obedient student and I am not surprise he made it to become great."

That was a teacher being proud of his student. But guess what would happen when a nurse say about her patient;

"He was my patient. I nursed him. He was diagnosed of Hernia. We worked on him and he recovered." Hell would break lose. It is unprofessional to do that in nursing. Your work has more restrictions and I believe that tells why it is unique and perhaps the noblest.

Well, I just want to encourage you with 21 thoughts I gathered from the globe. Some will inspire you, others will challenge you. Some will encourage you and still some may provoke you. I believe sometimes, you don't need to be inspired to make a change. You should be provoked to do it. No matter what these quotes will reflect in you, I trust they will bring a an inspiration that will enforce positive change on your career through you and in turn, a good reputation for the nursing profession.

Do enjoy them!

Nurses are the hospitality of the hospital – Carrie Latet

*Only nurses do stay with the patient 24 hours each day. No wonder they are the heart of the healthcare team for every hospital.*

The trained nurse has become one of the great blessings of humanity, taking a place besides the physician and the priest. – William Osler

*Society depends on the nurse for restoration and promotion of health. Since health is of a great concern, nurses are great assets a nation cannot do without.*

Nurses dispense comfort, compassion, and caring without even a prescription. – Val Saintsbury

*Sometimes, what a sick person needs is not Intravenous fluids, Intramuscular injections or oral medications. A cool, soothing comfort can lift them out of their symptoms. This is a nursing duty.*

The character of the nurse is just as important as the knowledge he or she possesses. – Carolyn Jarvis

*In as much as the knowledge of the nurse can help restore the health of the patient, her character is what will allow the patient to apply her knowledge on him. Character is essential just as knowledge.*

Our job as nurses is to cushion the sorrows and celebrate the job, every day, while we are just doing our jobs. – Christine Belle

*Even in sorrows and pains, a nurse isn't allowed to complain when there is job. The celebration of the nurse is not her complaints, but in the job.*

In engineering, you work on a broken machine that cannot question how hard you hit it with hammer. In nursing, you work on a broken person who can question how bitter your needle pricks. – Israelmore Ayivor

*Nurses feel what the patient feels. They don't take their pains for granted. Every procedure a nurse would perform, she wants to have an objective for it.*

Constant attention by a good nurse may just be just as important as a major operation by a surgeon. – Dag Hammarskjöld

*No careers is important than the other. It is how good you do it that makes it more important. A wonderful street sweeper is more important than an incompetent flight lieutenant.*

Apprehension, uncertainty, waiting, expectation, fear or surprise, do a patient more harm than any exertion – Florence Nightingale

*You don't leave a good mark when your care questionable. Unprofessionalism is a risky thing as far as nursing is concerned.*

Panic plays no part in training a nurse – Elizabeth Kenny

*Nursing goals are achieved with a full load of confidence. Nurses cannot do without the attitude of confidence. When*

*a nurse is trained with panic, she would not give out her best.*

…Nurses are the beating heart of our medical system. – Barack Obama

*When the heart stops, the body dies. When nurses go wayward, the life of the nation is just a matter of days away from tombs.*

To do what nobody else will do, in a way that nobody else can, in spite of all we go through; is to be a nurse. – Rawsi Williams

*Nurses hunger for excellence. There may be many options to do something, but the nurse strives to choose the best among the rest.*

Drugs are not always necessary; belief in recovery always is. – Norman Cousins

*Sometimes, people become sick when their true hopes leaves their bodies and wonder about. The duty of the nurse is to look for that hope wherever it is a fix it back where it belongs.*

People will forget what you said. They will forget what you did. But they will never forget how you made them feel. – Maya Angelou

*The name of the medicine you gave to the patient, he may forget in days to come, but the attitude you displayed to him, will never forgotten.*

It is not how much you do, but how much love you put in the doing. – Mother Theresa

*When you do what you love, you will love what you do. The bottom line is that there is no happiness in doing what you don't love. You will enjoy nursing if you love caring.*

Nursing is not for everyone. It takes a very strong, intelligent and compassionate person to take on the ills of the world with passion and purpose and work to maintain the health and well-being of the planet. No wonder we're exhausted at the end of the day. – Donna Wilk Cardillo

*Compassion is to feel and show love. By that attribute, the nurse extends his hands to lift up someone who needs her care irrespective of the person's status, creed, age or political affiliation.*

A nurse will always give us hope; an angel with a stethoscope. – Terri Guillemets

*Nurses look for the missing hope the patient needs, bring it and instill it back in place. They guard the patient 24 hours and that's why they are angels.*

Your employer is your employer and nursing is nursing. I understand you may not have been treated fairly by your employer, but I believe your patient did not contribute it. He is innocent. – Israelmore Ayivor

*The nurse should not let other people's actions interfere with the needs of the innocent patient under her care. Good health first, then other things follow.*

What inspires the nurse is likely to be the 90% of her inwardly-built compassion and 10% of her outward-earned compliments. – Israelmore Ayivor

*Let your job give you the motivation you need. When you allow this to happen, no one can frustrate you on the job.*

Sometimes we cry because can't save them all. God sometimes won't let us interfere when he calls. – Dawn Butler

*In all things remember you are an undertaker, doing the assignment of a mighty creator. When the creator calls a patient home, you have no question to ask.*

*Thank you for enjoying this book. Go, make nursing a great profession.*

REFERENCES

Awuah-Peasah, D, Sarfo, L.A, & Asamoah, F. (2013). The attitudes of student nurses toward clinical work. *International Journal of Nursing and Midwifery*. 5(2), pp. 22-27. DOI: 10.5897/ IJNM12.017

Bolton S.C ( 2001). Changing faces; nurses as emotional jugglers. *Sociology of Health & Illness*. 23(1), 85-100.

Calnan, M., & Rowe, R. (2005). Trust relations in new NHS: theoretical and methodological challenges. Retrieved from http://www.hsrc.ac.uk/current_research/research_projects/public_trust.html on 20/2/2017

Fauda, E.M., Sleem, W.F., & Mohammed, H.A. (2016): Nursing image as a profession and self-esteem among secondary school students in Dakalia governorate. *IOSR Journal of Nursing and Health Sciences*. 5(5), 65-75

George, J.B.(1995).*Nursing Theories: The Base for Professional Nursing Practice*(4th ed.).Norwalk, Connecticut: Appleton & Lange.

Ghana Registered Nurses Association (Facebook page). Retrieved from http://facebook.com/GRNAOfficial/posts/60503976289063 1 on 12 January, 2017.

Mok, E., & Chui, B. (2004). Nurse-Patient Relationships in palliative care. *Nurse-Patient Relationships in palliative care,* 48(5), 475-483.

Nurse-Patient Trust Relationship. An article by Nizar Belal Said. Retrieved from http://www.reesearchgate.net/.../ on 10th February, 2017.

Principle. Retrieved from www.vocabulary.com/dictionary/principle on 12/2/2017

Ogochukwu, P. (2009). *Will letters in harmattan*. Oracle Books Limited, Lagos: Nigeria.

Online Ethymology Dictionary. Retrieved from http://etymonline.com/index.php?term=nurse on 3rd January, 2017.

The Nurses' Pledge, The Midwives' Prayer. Retrieved from http://nursinginghana.com/nurses-pledge-midwives-player/ on 23/02/2017

Books by Israelmore Ayivor

- Mine Your Gold

- Rescue Your Visions

- Champions companion

- Get Busy and Grab it

- 30 Days to Better Life

- Leaders' Ladder

- Leaders' Watchwords

- 101 Keys to Everyday Passion

- 16 Mistakes Young Girls Make

- Take the Lead

- Grow Great & Giant

- Daily Drive 365

- Daily Motion 365

- The Great Hand Book of Quotes

- 21 Habits to Quit

- Creeds for Aspiring Achievers

- Dream Big (See your Bigger Picture)

- Shaping the Dream

- Believe and Achieve

- Michelangelo | Beethoven | Shakespeare

- You must be who God Said You must be

- You Can Rise

- Compass of Greatness

- 25 Questions to Ask your Potential Husband

- Become a Better You

- Leadership A to Z

- Let's Go to the Next Level

- Six Reasons You Are Afraid To Speak In Public

Grab your copy on Amazon:

http://www.amazon.com/author/IsraelmoreAyivor

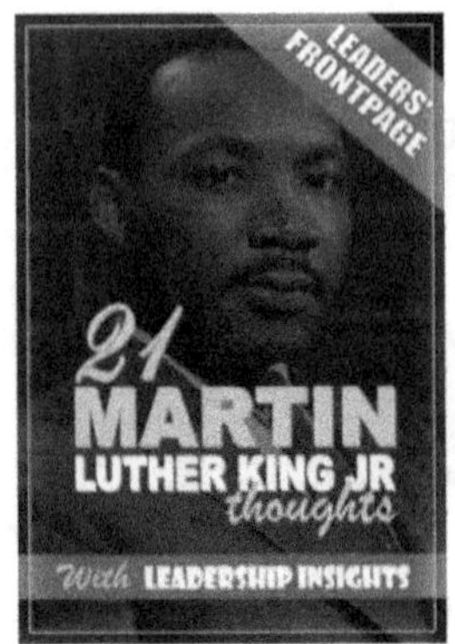

LEADERS' FRONTPAGE
21
MARTIN
LUTHER KING JR
thoughts
With LEADERSHIP INSIGHTS


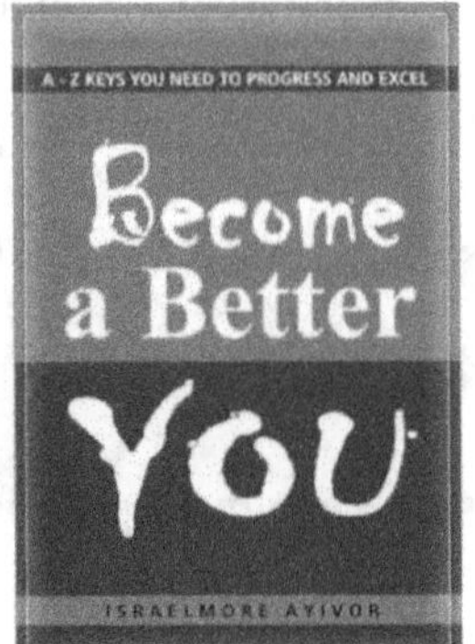

A - Z KEYS YOU NEED TO PROGRESS AND EXCEL
Become
a Better
YOU
ISRAELMORE AYIVOR


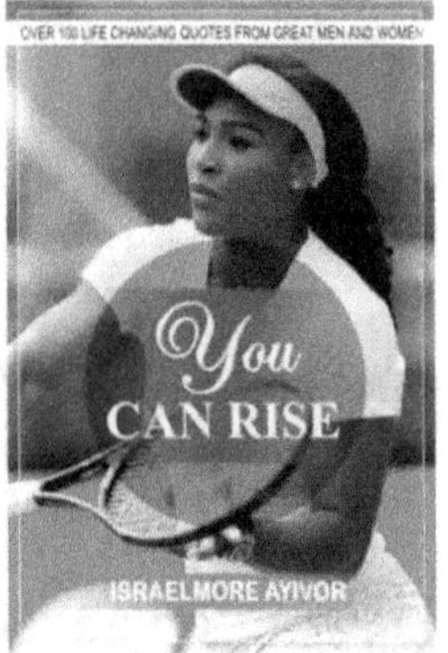

OVER 100 LIFE CHANGING QUOTES FROM GREAT MEN AND WOMEN
You
CAN RISE
ISRAELMORE AYIVOR


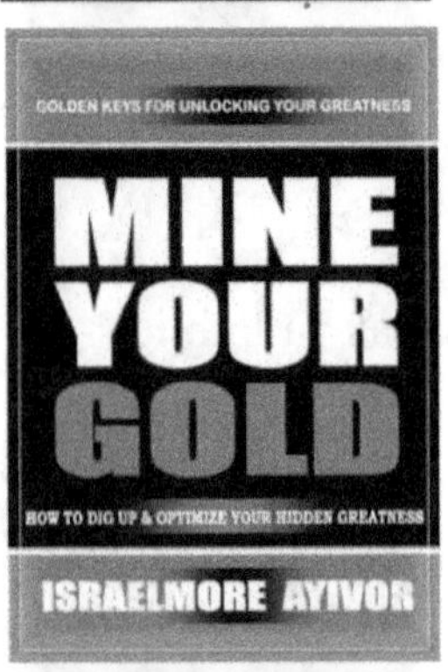

GOLDEN KEYS FOR UNLOCKING YOUR GREATNESS
MINE
YOUR
GOLD
HOW TO DIG UP & OPTIMIZE YOUR HIDDEN GREATNESS
ISRAELMORE AYIVOR


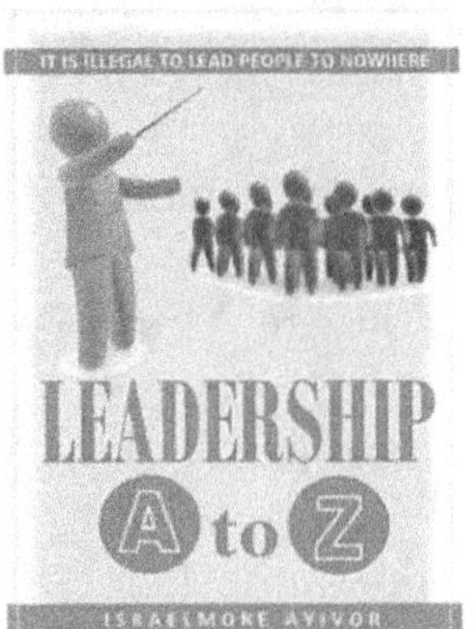

IT IS ILLEGAL TO LEAD PEOPLE TO NOWHERE
LEADERSHIP
A to Z
ISRAELMORE AYIVOR


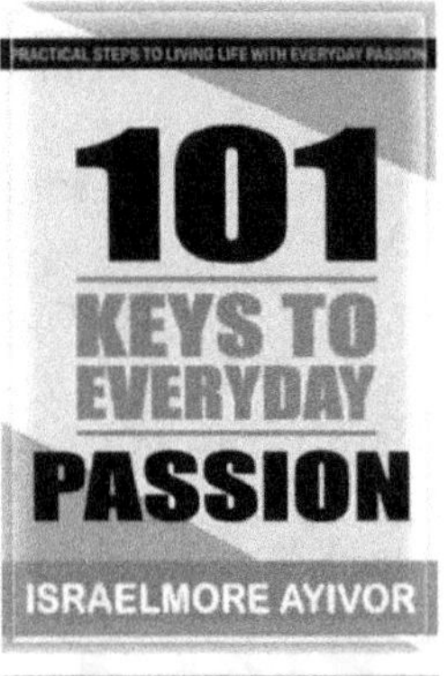

PRACTICAL STEPS TO LIVING LIFE WITH EVERYDAY PASSION
101
KEYS TO
EVERYDAY
PASSION
ISRAELMORE AYIVOR


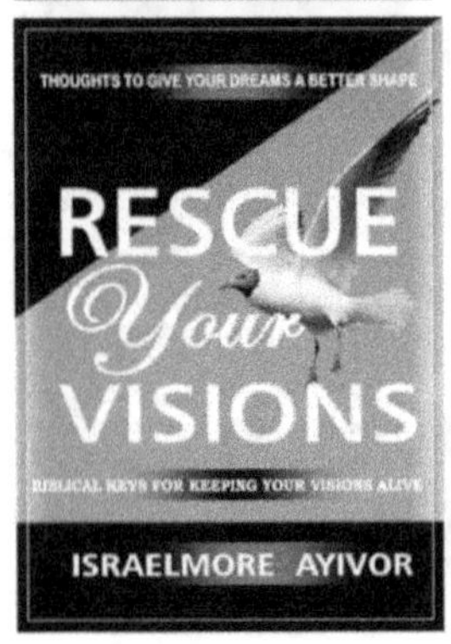

THOUGHTS TO GIVE YOUR DREAMS A BETTER SHAPE
RESCUE
Your
VISIONS
BIBLICAL KEYS FOR KEEPING YOUR VISIONS ALIVE
ISRAELMORE AYIVOR


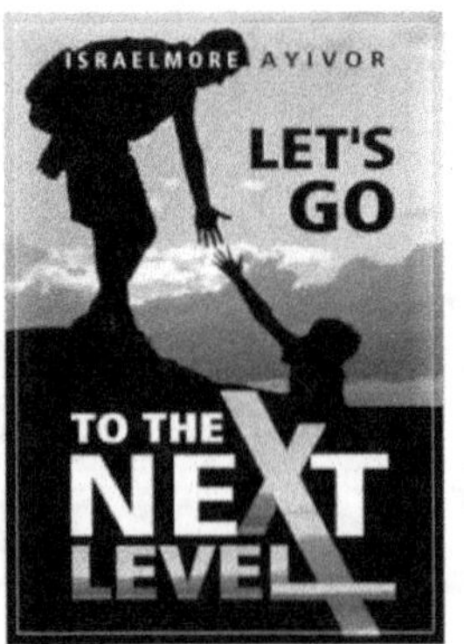

ISRAELMORE AYIVOR
LET'S
GO
TO THE
NEXT
LEVEL


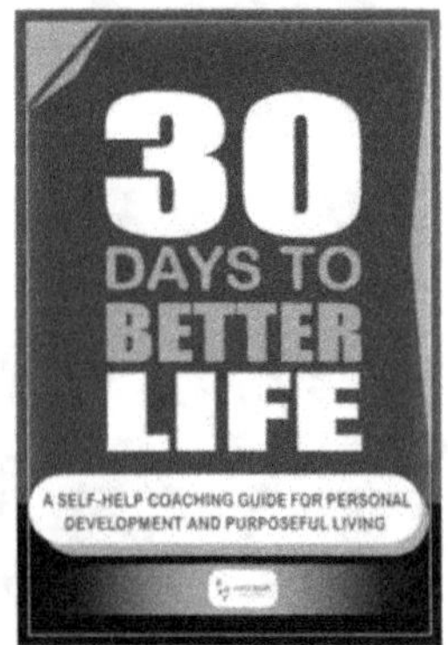

30
DAYS TO
BETTER
LIFE
A SELF-HELP COACHING GUIDE FOR PERSONAL
DEVELOPMENT AND PURPOSEFUL LIVING

# HIGHLY RECOMMENDED BOOK:

## YOU CAN RISE | Grab Your Copy Now

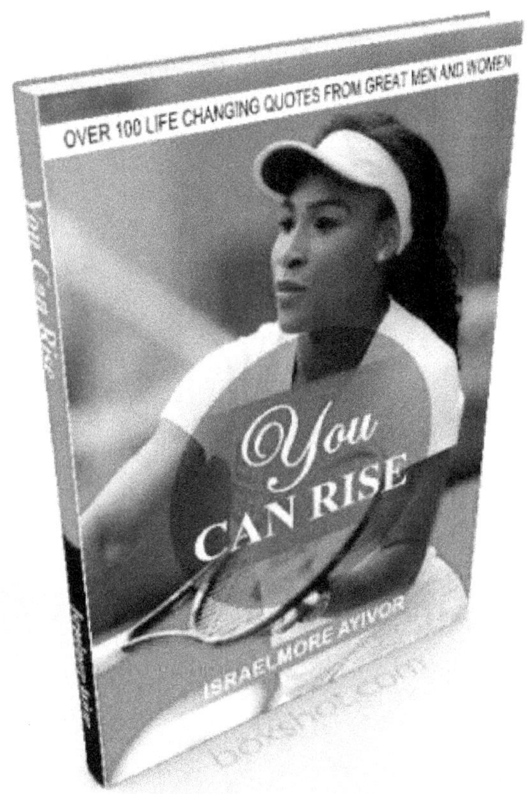


**<u>YOU CAN RISE</u>**

Your life-changing book! Strictly inspirational | Deeply
educational | Highly philosophical.